A Field Guide to
Medicinal and Useful Plants
of the
Upper Amazon

By

James L. Castner

Stephen L. Timme

James A. Duke

Published by
Feline Press
P.O. Box 357219
Gainesville, FL 32635 USA
e-mail: jlcastner@aol.com

A Field Guide To
Medicinal and Useful Plants
of the
Upper Amazon

By: James Lee Castner
      Stephen Lee Timme
      James Alan Duke

Published by:

Feline Press
P.O. Box 7219
Gainesville, FL
32605   USA

© 1998 by Feline Press, Inc.
Second Printing 2004
Printed in China

ISBN 0-9625150-7-8

Library of Congress
Catalog Card Number:
97-77509

Preface

In the past decade, there has been an intense effort on the part of developed nations to learn and record the knowledge of indigenous healers and *curanderos*, specifically with regards to medicinal and useful plants found in tropical forests. Sometimes the effort is motivated by purely financial reasons, such as the major pharmaceutical companies that are investing millions of dollars in tropical plant exploration. For others like Cox, Duke, Plotkin, Plowman, and Schultes, ethnobotanical research is a lifelong calling to quench a thirst for a certain kind of knowledge that may help mankind. Even the average person who doesn't feel this urge to go out and live among primitive tribes can at least share an appreciation and admiration for the dedication and accomplishments of those who have.

With the current interest in medicinal plants, rainforest conservation, and preserving the knowledge of indigenous peoples, it would seem natural that there would be a flood of books on the subject. However, we the authors found that there were actually a very limited number of works dealing with the topic. An even smaller number of the above were written for the general naturalist or layperson. We found none that was organized in the form of a photo-oriented field guide that could be carried along in the field and used to identify plants and compare their physical characteristics. It is this last unexploited literary 'niche' that we have tried to fill with: *A Field Guide To Medicinal And Useful Plants Of The Upper Amazon.*

Thousands of peolple visit the Amazon every year to see the rainforest with their own eyes. Many of these visitors have an interest in medicinal plants, as well as the important products and crops that are grown in the region. Although some books do exist treating certain aspects of these subjects, until now there was no easy to use guidebook for the layperson. In simple language and with clear color photos, the authors have tried to make it easy for anyone to recognize those plants with medicinal uses and with agricultural, economic, or cultural importance.

Unfortunately, there are more important plant species than there is room in a book to fill. The high cost of reproducing color artwork put a financial limitation on the number of color photos that could be used. However, with the collaboration of Peruvian shaman Don Antonio Montero Pisco, the expertise of medicinal plant expert Jim Duke, and the logistical support of Peter Jenson and Explorama Tours, the authors have tried to select the most important and representative plants of the Upper Amazon region for inclusion. Those visitors to the ACEER and Explornapo Camp outside of Iquitos, Peru, will find many of the plant species described on the following pages growing in the ReNuPeru Medicinal Plant Garden or along the Medicinal Plant Trail.

Acknowledgments

First, Stephen Timme and Jim Castner would like to recognize two people who represent different ends of the research spectrum and exemplify the cooperation and teamwork that can be achieved between different cultures. Don Antonio Montero Pisco is a *shaman* born and raised in the rainforests of the Peruvian Amazon. He learned about jungle plants from his grandparents, and has continued to add to his knowledge and practice traditional healing for the past 40 years. Two years ago, he began the development of a medicinal plant garden where he and his sons currently cultivate over 160 species of useful and medicinal herbs, shrubs, and trees. We thank Don Antonio for generously sharing his knowledge with us, and with the rest of the world.

Next, we would like to thank Dr. Jim Duke. Friend of the rainforest and medicinal plant expert extraordinaire, Jim is the 'yin' or complementary counterpart to Don Antonio as the 'yang'. Jim has devoted an entire professional career to investigating plants for their possible medicinal uses, especially with respect to anti-cancer agents. This work has required that he spend large amounts of time in places like the Darién in Panama and the Amazon of Peru, working with indigenous *curanderos*. Recently retired after 29 years with the U.S.D.A., Jim continues to work by lecturing and instructing people on the use of medicinal plants and how they affect our lives. Jim's generous donations initiated the creation of the ReNuPeru Medicinal Plant Garden and have made its maintenance and enlargement possible. With co-author Rodolfo Vasquez, Jim wrote the already classic *Amazonian Ethnobotanical Dictionary*, which is the best and most recent resource available for medicinal plants from the Peruvian Amazon. We used it constantly in preparing the current work. For year's we have benefitted from Jim's knowledge and enjoyed the friendship of this guitar-strumming gentleman who walks barefoot through the forest.

Third, we all would like to thank our friend Peter Jenson, the owner and originator of Explorama Tours. For over ten years, Peter has generously donated logistical support without which our work and many journeys to the rainforest would have been impossible. His support of our scientific research (SLT's dissertation work and JLC's Earthwatch work) has contributed directly to our professional enhancement and scientific expertise. A true supporter of education and the broadening of man's knowledge, Peter Jenson's help has allowed biologists, doctors, and even artists to have the opportunity to perform their chosen vocations in the rainforest. The creation and construction of the ACEER and Canopy Walkway was due in large part to his contributions and the logistical support provided by Explorama Tours. His professional and knowledgeable staff of Peruvian guides also receives our thanks.

Many of our colleagues have read portions of this manuscript and provided us with suggestions and corrections that have substantially improved the quality of this book. Others have generously provided us with access to plant specimens to photograph, allowed us to use their own photos, or helped us with our research or with logistical matters. For taking time from their busy schedules to do so we would like to thank: Michael Balick, Mark Blumenthal, Lynn Bohs, Christopher Campbell, Ara DerMarderosian, Paul Donahue, Hardy Eshbaugh, Robin Eskaof, Don Evans, Luis Gomez, Don Goodman, Dana Griffin, Gary Hartshorn, the Hopkins family, Walter Judd, Rose Karpenski, John Knaub, Bill Lorowitz, Andrew McRobb, Alan Meerow, Jorge Peña, Kent Perkins, Mark Plotkin, Hugh Popenoe, Pat Payne, Ghillean Prance, Peter Raven, Chris Rollins, April Rosenik, Larry Schokman, Linnea Smith, William Stern, Boyce Tankersley, Rodolfo Vasquez, and Mark Whitten. We would also like to thank both Samuel Minor and Cindy Ford for preparing line drawings for use in this work. Photographs not taken by James Castner or Stephen Timme are credited individually with the photographer's name.

Finally, we sadly recognize the wealth of information and boundless energy that was lost with the death of Al Gentry. His knowledge of tropical plant taxonomy was unsurpassed, and the extensive coverage in his *Woody Plants of South America* represents only a small part of it. As many times as the *Amazonian Ethnobotanical Dictionary* was consulted for medicinal information, so was Gentry's *Woody Plants* consulted for accurate taxonomic descriptions.

Dedications

I would like to recognize and thank my parents, Frank and Elizabeth Castner, for the education they have provided me with and the moral support they have extended to me throughout my life. They continue to be my most important teachers.   *James L. Castner*

I would like to thank Garland Owen for his continued encouragement; William E. and Esther M. Timme, who have never quite grasped my passion for plants; and lastly my family, Linda, Caleb and Zachary. Without their patience and understanding, my rainforest adventures would not have been possible.   *Stephe L. Timme*

I express my appreciation and my thanks to the Amazonian Rain Forest and to the employees of Explorama Lodge in Loreto, Peru, for all of the interesting lore I have learned.   *James A. Duke*

Warning - Disclaimer

This book is designed to provide information with regards to the subject matter covered. It is sold with the understanding that the publisher and the authors are not engaged in rendering medical advice or other related services. If medical or other expert assistance is required, the services of a competent doctor or physician should be sought.

It is not the purpose of this guide to reprint all the information that is otherwise available to the authors and/or publisher, but to complement, amplify, and supplement other texts. You are urged to read all the available material, and learn as much as possible about medicinal and useful plants. For more information, see the many references in the Bibliography.

Every effort has been made to make this guide as complete and as accurate as possible. However, there may be mistakes, both typographical and in content. Errors in translation from Spanish or Quechua to English may also have occurred. Therefore, this text should be used only as a general guide and resource, and not as the definitive source and reference work on medicinal and useful plants.

The purpose of this field guide is to educate and entertain in an informative, easy to use, and enjoyable manner. The authors and Feline Press shall have neither liability nor responsibility to any person or entity with respect to any loss or damage caused, or alleged to be caused, directly or indirectly, by the information contained in this book.

If you do not wish to be bound by the above, you may return this book to the publisher for a full refund.

Table of Contents

Leaf Margins

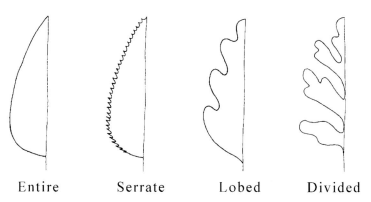

Entire   Serrate   Lobed   Divided

Leaf Venation

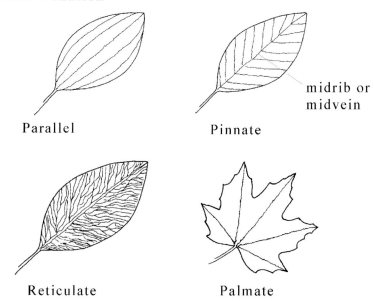

Parallel   Pinnate

midrib or midvein

Reticulate   Palmate

Leaf Arrangement

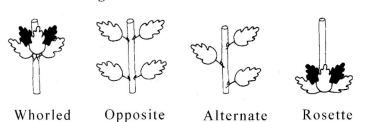

Whorled   Opposite   Alternate   Rosette

Leaf Blade Shapes

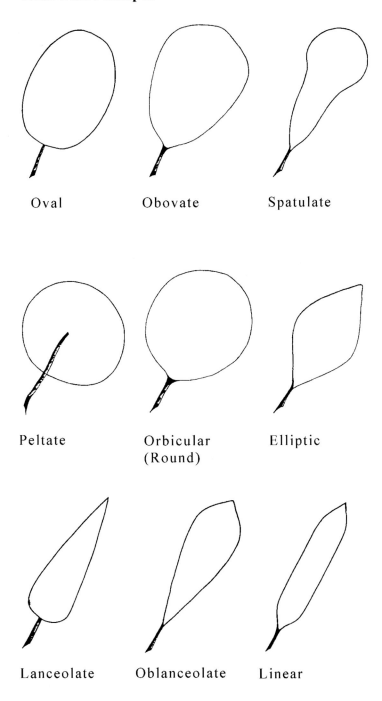

Oval · Obovate · Spatulate

Peltate · Orbicular (Round) · Elliptic

Lanceolate · Oblanceolate · Linear

4

Leaf Types

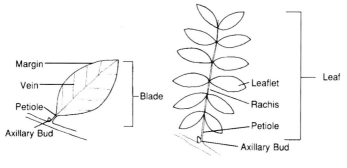

Margin
Vein
Petiole
Axillary Bud
Blade

Leaflet
Rachis
Petiole
Axillary Bud
Leaf

Simple   Compound

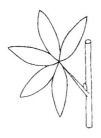

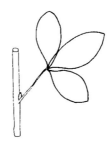

Palmately Compound   Ternately Compound
(Trifoliate)

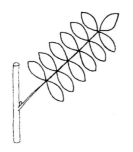

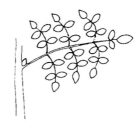

Pinnately Compound   Bipinnately Compound

Flower Anatomy

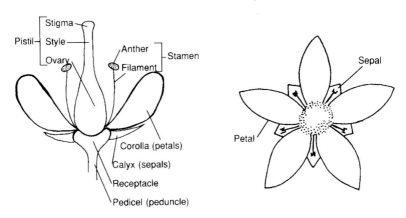

Flower Shapes

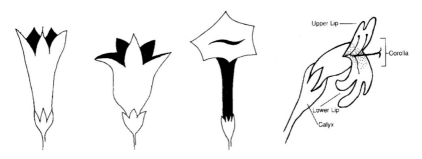

Tubular Campanulate Funnelform Bilabiate

Flower Types

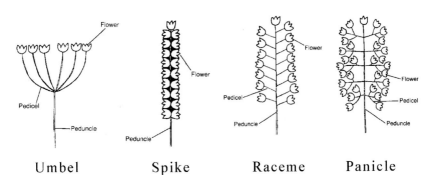

Umbel Spike Raceme Panicle

6

Glossary of Botanical Terms

aril - a fleshy seed coat or the fleshy appendage of a seed.

axil - the point between the axis of the stem and any part arising from it (leaf, branch, pedicel, etc.).

axillary - located at or arising from an axil.

blade - the expanded part of a leaf.

bract - a leaf-like structure located at the base of an inflorescence or flower.

calyx - all the sepals collectively.

campanulate - a flower that is bell-shaped.

capsule - a dry fruit composed of more than one carpel.

catkin - a spike or raceme of few to many flowers of the same sex.

cauliflory - bearing flowers directly from the trunk or branches.

cordate - heart-shaped (i.e. a leaf with lobes at its base).

corolla - the inner whorl of the perianth composed of the petals.

costapalmate - a palmate leaf with a petiole that extends through the blade as a midrib.

cyme - a compound determinate flat-topped inflorescence.

dehiscent - splitting opening at maturity (usually in reference to a dry fruit).

dentate - having teeth (usually in reference to the edge of a leaf blade).

dimorphic - consisting of two forms (i.e. a plant with two types of leaves).

dioecious - sexual condition in which pistillate (female) flowers are on one plant and staminate (male) flowers another. See monoecious.

drupe - a fleshy indehiscent fruit with a 'stone' or 'pit' that usually encloses a single seed.

druplet - a small drupe.

elliptic - broadest at the middle and narrowed towards the ends.

emarginate - in reference to leaves, a shallow notch at the apex.

fascicle - a cluster, generally referring to leaves or flowers.

follicle - a dry fruit with a single carpel that splits along one side.

funnelform - in the shape of a funnel, generally referring to a flower.

hemiepiphyte - a plant that initially grows by attaching via sucker-like roots to the stems or trunks of other plants which are used for support as it climbs to a level of sufficient light intensity, where it becomes epiphytic.

herb - a soft-stemmed plant; non-woody.

irregular - flowers in which similar parts are not the same size.

lanceolate - wide at the base and narrowed to a point at the apex.

leaflet - one of the divisions or segments of a compound leaf, each of which has its own blade and may or may not have a petiole.

midvein - the primary or central vein of a pinnately-veined leaf.

monocotyledon - plants that produce seeds with only one cotyledon (i.e. grasses).

monoecious - sexual condition in which pistillate (female) and staminate (male) flowers occur on the same plant. See dioecious.

multiple - a fruit resulting from the fusion of the ovaries of many flowers.

node - the part of a stem where one or more leaves are attached.

oblanceolate - a leaf shape that is wide at the apex and narrowed to the base.

oblong - a leaf approximately 2-4 times longer than wide with nearly parallel edges.

obovate - a leaf that is egg-shaped and attached at the narrow end.

pachycaul - a growth form characterized by foliage at the top of the stem or trunk giving an umbrella-shaped appearance.

palmate - diverging as lobes or veins from a common point at the base of a leaf.

panicle - inflorescence made up of loose flower clusters from a branched main axis.

pedicel - the stalk of a flower.

peduncle - the stalk of a flower cluster.

peltate - a leaf with the petiole attached near the center rather than at the base.

perianth - the calyx and corolla, collectively.

petal - an individual segment of the corolla of a flower.

petaloid - floral structures that are petal-like in form.

petiole - the stalk of a leaf.

pinna - a segment or division of a pinnately compound leaf.

pinnate - leaf venation with a central main vein and smaller diverging lateral veins, or a compound leaf with leaflets arranged on opposite sides of the axis or rachis.

pinnule - the smallest leaf-like segment of a multiply compound pinnate leaf.

pistil - the female reproductive structure of a flower.

pistillate - a flower that contains only the female reproductive organ.

prostrate - lying on the ground; the stems parallel or nearly so to the ground.

pulvinate - containing a pulvinus.

pulvinus - an enlarged area at the base of the petiole.

raceme - an inflorescence with stalked flowers on a long central axis.

rachis - the main axis of a compound leaf or inflorescence.

rhizome - a horizontal , underground, modified stem.

rhomboid - diamond-shaped or quadrangular.

rosette - a cluster of leaves near or at the base of the stem that radiate away from it.

scabrous - having a rough texture (like a cat's tongue).

scape - a leafless flowering stem (peduncle) that arises from the ground.

secondary vein - a vein that branches or diverges from the midvein of a leaf.

sepal - an individual segment of calyx; usually green, leaf-like, and enclosing bud.

serrate - leaf margin that is toothed, with the teeth pointing towards the apex.

sessile - without a stalk.

spadix - a spike densely packed with flowers so that the axis is not visible.

spathe - a bract or pair of bracts that surround an inflorescence.

spike - an inflorescence with non-stalked flowers attached to an unbranched stalk.

stamen - the male reproductive structure.

staminate - a flower that contains only the male reproductive organ or stamens.

stipule - a leaf-like appendage found at the base of some leaves, always in pairs.

strobilus - a cone that may contain male, female, or both reproductive structures.

subopposite - almost opposite.

trichome - a hair or hair-like structure.

trifoliate - three leaflets arising from a common point at the tip of the petiole.

tubular - a tube-shaped structure, typically referring to the corolla of a flower.

umbel - an inflorescence that is umbrella-shaped.

whorled - three or more structures arising from a node, typically referring to leaves.

Discussion of Selected Amazonian Plants

Ayahuasca or Soul Vine

Banisteriopsis caapi is a woody liana found in the tropical forest regions of northwest South America. It has many native names, the most well known of which are *ayahuasca, yagé*, and *caapi*. All of these names also refer to the hallucinogenic drink that is prepared from this plant. The large variety of recognized names reflects not only regional linguistical differences, but also the ability of indigenous tribes to distinguish between different varieties of the plant. The latter is something the botanist has been unable to do using traditional morphological taxonomic characteristics.

The drink *ayahuasca* is a powerful hallucinogen that has been employed by Amerindians in communal rituals which lead to shared visions. Shamans and *curanderos* also use *ayahuasca* in order to communicate with the spirit world in an effort to diagnose illnesses or seek answers to tribal crises. Two excellent works discussing the preparation and use of *ayahuasca* are *Vine Of The Soul* and *Wizard Of The Upper Amazon* (see Bibliography). In addition to the hallucinations induced by drinking *ayahuasca*, it also causes diarrhea and vomiting, and is in fact used as a purgative in many areas.

Ayahuasca is prepared in a number of ways, with each tribe using its own 'recipe' of ingredients. In many cases, the sole component is the bark of *B. caapi*, although 21 other plants have been identified as additives. The traditional method of preparation requires removing the bark from sections of the vine, boiling it in water, and drinking the resulting liquid. However, cold water infusions are also used and it is recorded that sometimes even the stems are chewed. Admixtures may be used to improve the flavor of the drink, but more commonly are included to lengthen and intensify the effect of the visions. With respect to the latter, two of the most widely used plants in Amazonia are *Psychotria viridis* (Rubiaceae) and *Diplopterys cabrerana* (Malpighiaceae). Antonio Montero Pisco reports using the following six *ayahuasca* additives: *Abuta grandifolia, Psychotria* sp., *Brugmansia suaveolens, Mansoa alliacea, Petiveria alliacea,* and a species of *Piper* called *guayusa*.

The psychoactive compounds of *B. caapi* have been identified as beta-carboline alkaloids called harmaline and harmine. They are structurally similar to and mimic the effects of the central nervous system neurotransmitter serotonin, resulting in the production of psychodelic visions. *P. viridis* and *D. cabrerana* both contain tryptamine alkaloids in their leaves. These compounds also provoke visions, but only when taken by smoking or as a snuff. If taken orally, an enzyme in the human digestive system deactivates them. However, the harmine and harmaline found in the *B. caapi* bark inhibit the action of this gut enzyme, which leads to a synergistic effect from the combination of all the ingredients that is profoundly more powerful and enduring.

Curare

Curare (pronounced *curaré* in Spanish) is a plant poison used by Indian groups throughout northern South America in hunting and killing game. It has become synonomous with arrow-poison and dart-poison due to its widespread use on the points of arrows and blowgun darts. The contents of curare and their preparation vary from region to region, a fact that made it very difficult for early explorers and medical researchers to obtain consistent samples of the substance. Historical accounts and information about the exploration and use of curare can be found in sections of *One River* and in *Earthly Goods* (see Bibliography).

The botanical contents of curare are derived primarily from tropical forest lianas in two genera. Vines in the genus *Chondrodendron* (Menispermaceae) are used in western Amazonia, while plants in the genus *Strychnos* (Loganiaceae) are used in most of Brazil and the Guianas. Typical preparation of curare uses the bark, although stems, and in some cases the seeds (with *Strychnos* spp.), have been used as well. One way to produce or extract curare requires scraping or rasping the bark from the source plants, pounding the bark, then filtering cold water through it in a rolled palm leaf. The dark filtered liquid is collected, heated, cooled, and reheated several times until it becomes thick and syrupy. The tips of the blowgun darts are dipped and rolled in this viscous, tarry substance then set by a fire to dry and harden. The efficacy of the poison and the duration of its potency will vary with the manner of preparation and the species of plants from which it was extracted.

A variety of both botanical and animal additives may be used when making curare. Ingredients vary regionally, and even from person to person. Antonio Montero Pisco lists the following plant additions: *Abuta grandifolia, Brunfelsia grandiflora*, and *Brugmansia suaveolens*. Other records have included *Tetrapterys mucronata* and *Anthodiscus obovatus*. Extracts are used from the small, brightly colored frogs in the genus *Dendrobates* (known as dart-poison frogs), which contain similar chemicals to the active compounds found in the source plants. In addition, venom from the large stinging ants belonging to the genus *Paraponera* may also be used.

The effect of curare is the result of several alkaloids present. Tubocurarine is derived from *Chondrodendron* spp., while species of *Strychnos* yield strychnine, curarine, and toucine. These inhibit neuromuscular activity by blocking the neurotransmitter acetylcholine. This prevents nerve impulses from reaching the muscles which results in paralysis and eventual death due to respiratory failure. Since curare does not affect heart action, it found widespread applications in the medical world as a muscle relaxant. Its use greatly decreased the amount of anesthesia necessary, significantly lowering the negative side effects and associated risks. It also made possible delicate operations where complete muscle relaxation was essential.

Coca

Perhaps no other plant with South American origins is as well known throughout the world as is coca, from which the drug cocaine is produced. Linguistics can be confusing regarding this plant and its derivatives. Coca refers to the plants in the genus *Erythroxylon* (also spelled *Erythroxylum*) (Erythroxylaceae) and to their leaves. Cocaine refers to one of the alkaloids contained in the coca leaves, and to the drug containing this compound that is so often taken and abused. The most common form of the drug is a hydrochloride salt known as coke. *Cacao* refers to the tree (*Theobroma cacao*) from which chocolate or cocoa is produced. *Coco* is the Spanish word for coconut, a product harvested from the coconut tree (*Cocos nucifera*).

Cocaine is considered one of the scourge drugs of developed countries, yet coca leaves have been an integral and beneficial part of Indian cultures in the Andes for thousands of years. It was considered a sacred plant by the Incas, who buried bags of leaves alongside their dead. Coca leaves not only help mountain inhabitants withstand the rigors of a high altitude existence by acting as a mild stimulant and hunger depressant, but also have nutritional value. The leaves contain more calcium than any other edible plant, which is an important dietary factor in the Andes where dairy products are seldom consumed. Coca leaves are also high in certain vitamins and minerals, as well as in carbohydrates, protein, fiber, and calories. Recent studies show that they may also aid in the regulation of glucose metabolism. An entire chapter in the book *One River* is devoted to the treatment of coca.

Traditional use of coca by Amerindians, such as the ancient Incas, usually involves the chewing of the leaves. Two commonly cultivated species are *E. coca* and *E. novogranatense*. Once the leaves are harvested or picked, they are dried, but not to the point of becoming brittle. Several leaves are taken in the mouth at a time and chewed. They are typically dipped in or taken with lime, usually in the form of ash produced by burning and pounding the leaves of other plants. Lime facilitates the release of the alkaloids from the coca leaves and their absorption. It is often carried in a separate bag or container. The chewed mass of leaves or 'quid' is maintained between the cheek and gum much in the same way chewing tobacco is used. Coca taken in this way helps to alleviate hunger and gives stamina, while producing a slight feeling of euphoria.

The chemical basis of the effects produced by coca usage are related to the central nervous system neurotransmitter dopamine and the pleasure centers of the brain. The release of dopamine from nerve cells in the brain causes feelings of pleasure and euphoria. Shortly after its release, dopamine is normally reabsorbed back into the nerve cell. The alkaloid cocaine blocks the reabsorption of dopamine, extending the pleasurable feelings caused by their original release.

Coca has resulted in distinct benefits to the developed world. Early investigations into cocaine and its derivatives showed that they produced a numbing or deadening sensation. Further experimentation led to cocaine's widespread use as a local anesthetic, especially in eye, ear, nose, and throat surgery. Although cocaine itself is now seldom used, chemically similar synthetic drugs such as novocaine and lidocaine have been developed and are used extensively. They are often administered in situations requiring dental surgery or the introduction of 'stitches' to close wounds.

Shortly after it was first isolated, cocaine was adopted as a treatment for morphine and alcohol dependencies, headaches, and even depression. It became increasingly popular and began to be used in a number of tonics, wines, and other beverages. The most famous evolved from an early medicine into a soft drink which used the extract of kola nuts and was called Coca Cola. Modern ingredients no longer permit the inclusion of cocaine.

Virola

Virola is a genus of small to medium-size trees in the Neotropics. In northern South America, several species are used to manufacture a hallucinogenic powder that is commonly taken as a snuff, but is also consumed in the form of pellets made from a paste. Amerindians use the inner bark of virola trees, preparing it in a manner similar to that described for curare. The final product is often blown forcefully into the user's sinuses by a partner using a long grass tube. It is also self-administered by means of V-shaped bird bones set in a reservoir of the snuff. The psychoactive compounds are tryptamines.

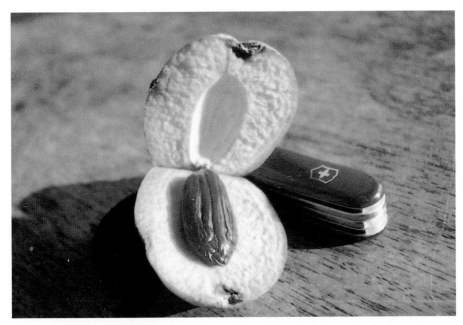

An opened virola fruit showing the characteristic red aril. (Photo by Gary Hartshorn)

Citation Abbreviations

The following is a list of citation abbreviations that were used throughout this book. The complete bibliographic citation for each of the abbreviations can be found in the Bibliography (page 135). To minimize confusion, the same abbreviations as those found in the *Amazonian Ethnobotanical Dictionary* were used in most cases.

AAB = Arvigo and Balick
AED = Amazonian Ethnobotanical Dictionary
AHG = Alwyn H. Gentry (Publications & Personal Communications)
AL = Anna Lewington
AMP = Antonio Montero Pisco (Personal Communications)
AYA = Ayala, Flore F.
BDS = Branch and DaSilva
CAA = Cayon and Aristizabal
CFNA = Cultivo de Frutales Nativos Amazónicos
DAT = Denevan and Tracy
DAW = Duke and Wain
ESG = Gómez, Eduardo S.
FOR = Forero, P.L.E.
GMJ = Grenand, Moretti, and Jacquemin
HGB = Henderson, Galeano, and Bernal
JAD = James A. Duke (Personal Communications & Observations)
MC = Castleman, Michael
MJB = Balick, M.J.
NIC = Maxwell, Nicole
PEA = Perez-Arbelaez, E.
POV = Poveda, L.J.
RAR = Rutter, R.A.
RVM = Vasquez Martinez, Rodolfo
SAO = Simpson and Ogorzaly
SAR = Schultes and Raffauf
SOU = Soukup, J.
SWPT = Smith, Williams, Plucknett, and Talbot
TBC = Croat, Thomas B.
TRA = Robineau, L.
VDF = Feo, Vincent de

Abuta
Motelo Sanango

Latin Name: *Abuta grandifolia* (Mart.) Sandwith.
Menispermaceae: Moonseed Family

Description: The example of abuta observed was growing as a small bush about a meter high. The simple, alternate, entire leaves range from 15cm long by 5cm wide to 45cm long by 15cm wide. They are borne on a petiole 4-12cm long, and that is twisted, wiry, and expanded at its apex where it joins the leaf. The leaves terminate in a blunt obvious drip-tip at least a centimeter in length. There are three longitudinal subparallel veins dividing the leaf into four sections, the outer two being the smallest. At a glance, the leaves are similar in appearance to those of the family Melastomataceae, but the latter are oppositely arranged. Secondary veins are less obvious, parallel to one another and intersect the longitudinal veins at right angles. The fruits are single seeds about 2-3cm long, and covered with a fleshy coating (= drupes).

Uses: According to SAR, abuta has attained widespread use throughout the Amazon by indigenous peoples as an ingredient in the preparation of arrow-poisons and dart-poisons used in hunting. Either extracts of the bark or raspings of the root may be mixed with species of *Chondrodendron* (page 36) and *Strychnos* (page 121) to produce a potent curare. Other uses are to treat snakebite, infected eyes, and as a tonic during childbirth or to a nervous child (SAR). Abuta in various forms is used for fever, toothaches, malaria, rheumatism, as an aphrodisiac, and to treat sterility in women (AED).

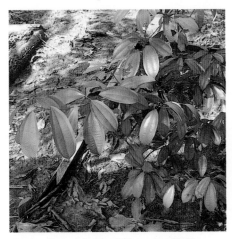

Fig. 1   Growth habit of *Abuta grandifolia*.

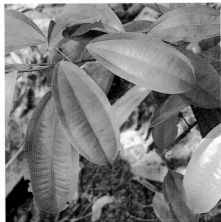

Fig. 2   The distinctive three-veined leaf of *Abuta grandifolia*.

Cashew
Cashu, Marañón

Latin Name: *Anacardium occidentale* L.
Anacardiaceae: Poison Ivy or Sumac Family

Description:　Cashew is grown throughout the tropical regions of the world, but is native to Brazil. It ranges from a small to medium-sized tree, with simple, alternate, broadly oval leaves that are borne on a short petiole. The mature leaves are 10-15cm long and 5-6cm wide. The midrib and secondary venation are a distinctive yellow against a dark green background, except for new leaves which may be copper-colored. The small blossoms are clustered at the tips of the branches and white while young, but turning pink and red with age. They are about one centimeter long and about a centimeter in diameter. The fruit is very distinctive consisting of a large fleshy, juicy portion (pedicel) called a 'cashew apple', and a smaller C-shaped fruit proper from which the edible nut is extracted. The cashew apple is about the size and shape of a bell pepper and turns yellow or red at maturity. The bark produces a yellow resin.

Uses:　Cashews are grown or harvested for a variety of reasons, including the commercial production of cashew nuts which are consumed primarily in the industrialized nations of the world. Although the roasted seeds or nuts are edible and a high-priced commodity in their final state, the latex from the non-roasted fruit is a vesicant and toxic. In the Third World, cashew consumption most often refers to the 'apple', which can be eaten fresh or squeezed for

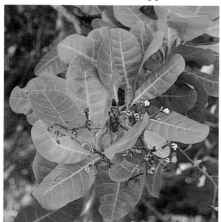

Fig. 3　Typical leaf growth of a cashew tree.

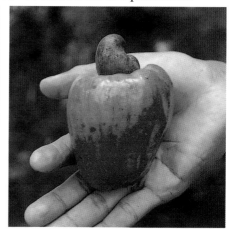

Fig. 4　The distinctive fruit of the cashew tree consists of the fleshy 'apple' and the hard brown fruit proper containing the cashew nut.

its juice. The juice is high in Vitamin C, and is bottled and consumed in great quantities in Brazil. The juice may also be fermented to make a cashew wine or cashew brandy. The liquid (cardol) derived from the cashew nut shell has been used to produce varnishes, lacquers, and preservatives (SWPT).

Some Indian groups make a brew from the cashew bark and take it to treat diarrhea, while others use it as a contraceptive (SAR) or as an astringent (AED). The nut shell latex has been used to treat maladies ranging from warts to scurvy to ringworm. Leaf infusions have been used both for toothache and diarrhea (AED).

The cultivation of cashew has spread from Brazil and the New World and is cosmopolitan throughout the tropics. Brazil and India are the major producers of cashew. Cashew trees are drought tolerant and do well in poor sandy soils, making them an excellent agricultural choice in some poorly managed tropical areas. (SWPT)

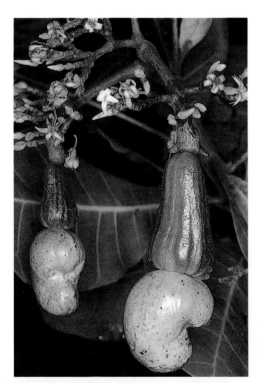

Fig. 5   Developing cashew fruits and flowers. Note how the nut portion is larger than the 'apple' portion at this point in the fruit development.

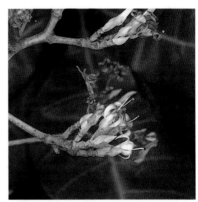

Fig. 6   Close up of a cluster of cashew flowers.

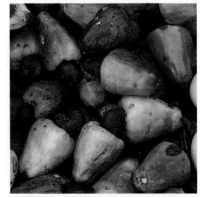

Fig. 7   Ripe cashew 'apples' for sale in the Belem market in Iquitos, Peru.

Pineapple
Piña

Latin Name: *Ananas comosus* L.
Bromeliaceae: Bromeliad or Pineapple Family

Description: Most species in this family grow as epiphytes using the trunks and branches of trees for support, however the pineapple grows in soil as a terrestrial bromeliad. Indigenous to South America, it is a perennial herb that grows in a rosette of long slender rigid pointed strap-like leaves with serrated edges. The plant may reach a height of a meter with a diameter that is slightly larger. The edible pineapple itself is a multiple fruit that grows at the top of a sturdy stalk. The name 'pine apple' was coined by Europeans that thought the fruit resembled a pine cone. Green while developing, it turns yellow-brown when ripe while increasing in size up to 45cm.

Uses: Pineapples have been cultivated in the Neotropics since the 1500's. It is now grown throughout the world. The white or yellow internal portion of the fruit is extremely sweet and juicy. It is sold and exported commercially for consumption raw, in preserves, as juice, in salads, in desserts, and canned. Fibers from the leaves have been used to make fine shirts and clothing. A protein-degrading enzyme (bromelain) is extracted from the stems and used commercially as a meat tenderizer, while also being investigated in blood clot-dissolving therapy. Indigenous peoples use pineapple juice to aid in digestion and to help heal wounds. Juice of the immature fruit is used as an abortive (SAR) and as a vermifuge (AED).

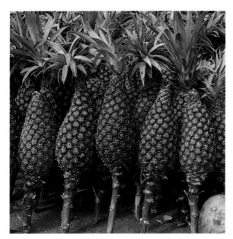

Fig. 8   Pineapple fruit (still attached to the stalk) in the Belem market in Iquitos, Peru.

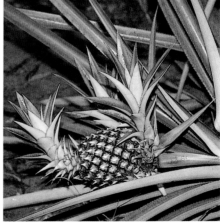

Fig. 9   Pineapple, a terrestrial bromeliad, usually grows upright but sometimes lodges.

Dye Plant
Puca Panga

Latin Name: *Arrabidaea chica* (HBK) Verlot.
Bignoniaceae: Trumpet Vine or Catalpa Family

Description: Dye plant is a sprawling, climbing vine when young that matures into a woody liana. It belongs to the most common vine genus in the trumpet vine family. The leaves are compound and oppositely arranged, and may be found with two or three leaflets on the same plant. The leaflets are 3-5cm wide by 15-18cm long, slender, and lanceolate. The leaf petioles are 12-15cm long and slightly swollen at the base where they connect to the stem. In cases where the leaves are trifoliate, the petiole of the central leaflet is noticeably longer than the others. Simple tendrils are present with some leaves. The fruits are linear and flat.

Uses: The liquid extracted from the crushed leaves is used to paint ceramics, as well as to dye woven materials and fibers. It is sometimes prepared in conjunction with the juice of the fruits of *Renealmia alpinia* (page 108) (AED). The liquid is also used as a face and body paint and may result in a red or black color (SAR). An extract of the leaves in water is believed to increase the blood supply and is used to treat anemia and paleness (AMP). (Perhaps a Doctrine of Signatures use based on the red dye that is produced?) Various Indian groups use a leaf infusion as an eye bath to treat conjunctivitis, and chew leaves to blacken the teeth (SAR). The leaves may also be used as an antiinflammatory agent (AED).

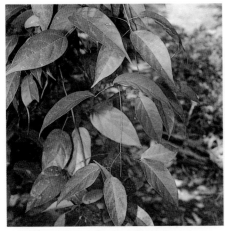

Fig. 10   Foliage of a young dye plant
(*Arrabidaea chica*), with mostly bifoliate leaves.

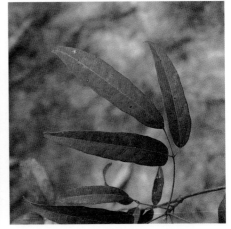

Fig. 11   Compound leaf of the dye plant
(*Arrabidaea chica*) showing a trifoliate leaf.

Breadfruit
Pan del Árbol

Latin Name: *Artocarpus altilis* (Park.) Fosb.
Moraceae: Fig or Mulberry Family

Description: The breadfruit tree is unmistakable due to its large size, and distinctive huge leaves and fruits. The broad leaves may reach 60cm in length, and have deep sinuses giving them a finger-like appearance on the edge. The inflorescence is long (25-40cm), yellow, and phallic-shaped and often attracts many bees. The fruits are round to oval with a spiny texture, light green in color, and may weigh from 1-5 kilograms. This evergreen tree grows wild in New Guinea and is indigenous to the geographical area that includes New Guinea, the Moluccas, and the Philippines.

Uses: The breadfruit tree is cultivated primarily for its edible fruit, which most of us recognize at least by name due to its role in British history in connection with the *HMS Bounty* and Captain Bligh. Beneath the thin spiny outer skin of the fruit is a pulpy yellow material that can be prepared by boiling, frying, baking, or roasting. The fruits are high in carbohydrates and a dietary staple in areas of the Pacific and Southeast Asia. Some indigenous peoples use the latex of the tree to caulk boats as well as a treatment for rheumatism (SWPT). In the Amazon Basin, treatments derived from the breadfruit tree are used for alleviating pain in connection with burns, diabetes, gout, and rheumatism (AED). In other parts of the world, breadfruit remedies are used to treat asthma, bronchitis, and coughs (SWPT).

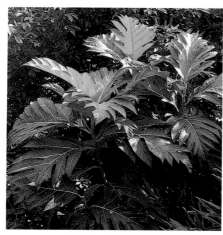

Fig. 12   The large broad finger-like evergreen leaves of the breadfruit tree.

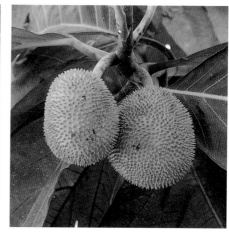

Fig. 13   Fruits of the breadfruit tree.

Tropical Milkweed
Flor de Muerto

Latin Name: *Asclepias curassavica* L.
Apocynaceae: Dogbane Family

Description: Known as blood flower in English and as *benzenyuco* or *pucasisa* in Spanish, this plant was formerly placed in the family Asclepiadaceae. It is an herb, and has the typical milky latex that is characteristic of the genus *Asclepias*. The leaves are opposite, or occasionally arranged in whorls of three, and have short petioles. Leaves usually range from 6-10cm long and 2-3cm wide. They are lanceolate with entire margins. The inflorescence is an umbel with numerous flowers that have five reddish to orange petals and yellow hoods. Individual flowers are about 1cm by 1cm in size. The fruit is a slender follicle about 8-12cm long that splits along one side to release the fluffy, wind-dispersed seeds. The silky nature of the material attached to the seed accounts for the Spanish name *flor de seda* (silk flower).

Uses: Indigenous groups use the milky latex for relief of toothaches or for the extraction of decayed teeth (SAR, RVM). The latex is also mixed with water as a treatment for intestinal parasites (SAR). The flowers are used to help stop bleeding and to treat diarrhea, while the ground roots are used to induce vomiting (AED). A shoot decoction is used as eyedrops for infections (GMJ). The leaves have been used to treat wounds, while the latex has also been used as a rat poison (AED). Note: The latex of this plant is considered extremely poisonous and contains various heart poisons (cardiac glycosides).

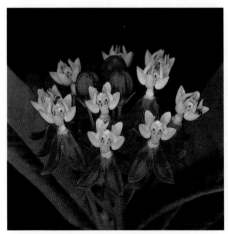

Fig. 14   The distinctive umbel of red and yellow flowers of tropical milkweed.

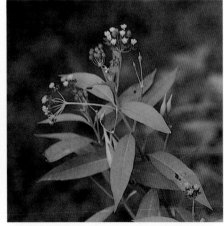

Fig. 15   Flowers, leaves, and developing seed pods of the tropical milkweed or blood flower.

Star Fruit
Carambola

Latin Name: *Averrhoa carambola* (Sw.) Beauv.
Oxalidaceae: Wood Sorrel Family

Description: This Asian fruit tree should not be confused with the native neotropical *Clusia rosea* (page 39), which is also called star fruit. Carambola trees seldom exceed ten meters in height. They have alternate odd pinnately compound leaves that range 20-24cm in length. The lanceolate leaflets have drip-tips and vary in number from 7-15 (TBC). They are asymmetrical and range from 3cm long by 2cm wide at the base to 7cm long by 3cm wide at the tip. The small flowers are reddish and usually occur on twigs below leaves or on old wood. The distinctive waxy appearing fruit is unmistakable with five longitudinal ribs. When cut in cross-section it resembles a star. It is light green at first, maturing to yellow or orange and ranging from 7-12cm long by 4-6cm wide. The fruits may occur singly or hang in clusters, borne on weak stalks of 2-5cm length. This tree often bears dense quantities of fruits.

Uses: This tree is widely cultivated in the tropics for its fruit which can be eaten raw, used as a juice, or processed into jellies or marmalade.

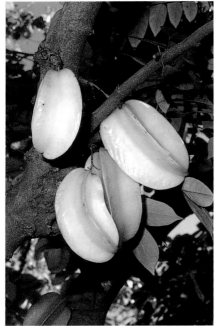

Fig. 16   The fruit of the star fruit tree (*Averrhoa carambola*).

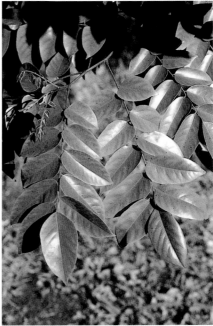

Fig. 17   The leaf of a star fruit tree (*Averrhoa carambola*).

Soul Vine
Ayahuasca, Yagé

Latin Name: *Banisteriopsis caapi* (Spruce ex Griseb.) Morton
Malpighiaceae: Malpighia Family

Description: Soul vine is a plant that has more than fifty vernacular names in Spanish in Amazonia where it is used. It is a liana with simple opposite leaves that have entire margins. The leaves terminate in a point that may or may not be extended into a drip-tip. Mature leaves are approximately 10-12cm long and 6-8cm wide. Secondary veins are alternate and do not quite reach the leaf edge. The pink or yellow flowers are about two centimeters in diameter and occur in clusters, arising from the space between the leaf petiole and the stem. Each has five petals with a fringe-like margin and narrow stalk at its base.

Uses: The main use of soul vine is as a hallucinogenic drink (*ayahuasca*) that is made from the bark of the plant. Several other plant species are used as additives when preparing the brew (see Discussion, page 8). It has a long history of use and importance in various ceremonies led by tribal shamans and *ayahuasqueros*. Soul vine has been used as a 'cure all' for many kinds of medical problems. It is commonly used within the Amazon region as a laxative and emetic (AED). Shamans are believed to be able to cure various ailments through communication with the spirit world, which is reached while under the effects of the drug. Much has been written about the use of *ayahuasca* and its powers (see Bibliography).

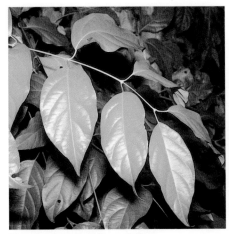

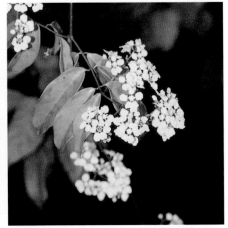

Fig. 18 Leaves of the soul vine.

Fig. 19 A cluster of distinctive soul vine flowers.

Monkey Ladder
Escalera de Mono

Latin Name: *Bauhinia guianensis* **Aubl.**
Fabaceae: Pea or Bean Family

Description: The vines known as monkey ladders are among the easiest of forest lianas to identify, both due to their unusual growth habit and their foliage. The woody stem of the vine itself tends to be flattened and wavy, sometimes with deep depressions within the body of the stem. This gives it the appearance of steps and hence the name 'monkey ladder'. The degree of curviness of the stem varies and at times the stem may split or divide. The leaves are simple and alternate, rounded at the base but deeply split down the middle with the tip of each half pronounced into a point. This medial split may extend anywhere from one third to almost the entire distance to the petiole. The leaf shape, when the split is extensive, resembles a cow's hoof and has resulted in the Spanish name *pata de vaca*. Mature leaves are 10-12cm long by 8-10cm wide, with a 3-5cm long petiole. New leaves are tightly folded in half and may be reddish in color. The venation is palmate, with several subparallel longitudinal veins extending from the leaf base to the tip on each side. Some leaves have simple tendrils associated with them.

Uses: In different Indian tribes, the stems are used to treat kidney diseases while the seeds are employed as diuretics (SAR). An extract of the root is also used in the treatment of amoebic diseases (BDS). Some people cut interesting-looking sections of the vine and use them for decorations.

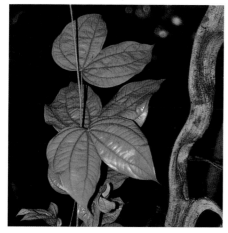 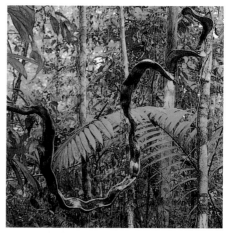

Fig. 20   Deeply cleft leaves and curvy stem of the monkey ladder vine.

Fig. 21   An undulating section of the forest liana known as monkey ladder.

Nispero
Níspero

Latin Name: *Bellucia* sp.
Melastomataceae: Melastome Family

Description: The trees of this genus are found in areas of secondary forest. Nispero seldom gets more than 12-15 meters high. The branches are squarish and angular, with the leaves clustered towards the ends. The large leaves are simple, opposite, and have entire margins. They are leathery, slightly wavy, and may measure 25-30cm long by 15-20cm wide. The venation is typical of that in melastomes, with three large obvious longitudinal veins starting above the leaf base and continuing to the tip. These divide the leaf into four easily visible sections. The secondary veins for the most part originate nearly perpendicular to the longitudinal veins. The flowers are large, white, and borne along the branches. The apple-scented fruit are tulip-shaped in profile, green while developing turning yellow at maturity. The open, flattened posterior end is six-sided, about 3-4cm in diameter, and has a brown ring surrounded by six roughly triangular green-yellow segments. The fruit is approximately 3-4cm long and borne on a slender stalk of roughly the same length.

Uses: The bark of nispero is mixed with water to form a brew given to women who have recently had babies, supposedly to serve as an internal vaginal wash and to promote healing (AMP). Green fruits may also be used. Some indigenous groups use the fruit to treat worms, the crushed leaves topically for sprains, and the juice from the stem for dyeing gourds (SAR).

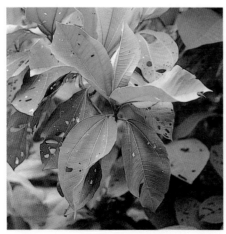

Fig. 22   A cluster of leaves of *nispero*.

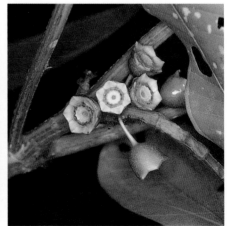

Fig. 23   A bunch of developing *níspero* fruits.

Brazil Nut
Castaña

Latin Name: *Bertholletia excelsa* **HBK.**
Lecythidaceae: Brazil Nut Family

Description: Brazil nut trees are found in the Amazon Basin with their greatest concentrations in southeast Peru, and northern Brazil, and Bolivia. It is an emergent species and one of the largest rainforest trees, sometimes reaching a height of 40-45 meters at maturity. It has a large straight trunk with dark bark that proceeds nearly unbroken until the top where the crown spreads out. The simple leaves are large and leathery, generally oval-shaped with entire margins, borne on short petioles and terminating in short points. The pale yellow flowers are marble-sized and fall quickly if not fertilized. Pollination is by several large bee species that are capable of forcing their way through the rigid flower petals. The fruit is a roundish, woody capsule, extremely thick, and ranging in size from 15-30cm in diameter. The fruits usually contain from 12-25 hard angular seeds which are the Brazil nuts of commerce.

Uses: Brazil nuts are extracted from wild trees as a high value export crop. They are also consumed by indigenous peoples who sometimes grate them and add them to a mixture of manioc flour. The seeds have an extremely high oil content and can literally be burned as vegetative candles (SWPT). When extracted, Brazil nut oil can be used in lamps, soap, or for cooking. The wood of the tree itself is prized due to its weather-resistant qualities (SWPT). A brew from the bark is used by some to treat liver diseases (SAR).

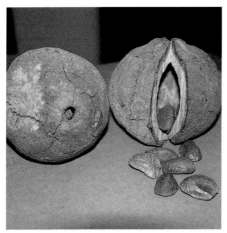 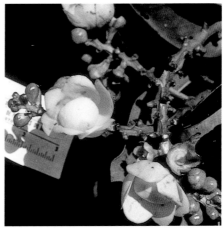

Fig. 24   Brazil nut fruits with nuts that have been extracted from the fruit capsule.

Fig. 25   Flowers of the Brazil nut tree. (Photo by Ghillean Prance)

Spanish Needles
Amor Seco

Latin Name: *Bidens alba* (L.) A. DC.
Asteraceae: Sunflower Family

Description: Spanish needles is a weedy upright herb, often found in disturbed areas and along trails or roadsides where it typically grows no more than two meters high. It has a square stem and branches with opposite, compound leaves that range from 6-20cm in length. The majority of leaves have three leaflets, although some have five and others only one. On the average trifoliate compound leaf, all the leaflets are lanceolate and pointed with regular dentate edges. The middle/terminal leaflet is largest, ranging from 8-9cm long by 3-3.5cm wide. The lateral leaflets are asymmetrical at their base, 6-7cm long by 2.5-3cm wide, and have a narrow constriction of 5mm or less that attaches to the rachis. The typical aster flower is 2-2.5cm in diameter with 5-7 white ray florets surrounding a yellow center of disk florets that is about 3-5mm in diameter. The flowers are borne on 2-3cm long stalks from the leaf axils and may occur singly or in small groups. The slender seeds are 6-8mm long by 1mm wide and have two prongs 2-3mm long at the end. They are held tightly together in a compact cylindrical bundle while green and immature, but turn brown with age, spreading like the seeds on a dandelion head.

Uses: Spanish needles is prepared in a variety of ways to treat an array of medical problems. These include mouth sores, sore throat, dysentery, chills (AED); toothache and headache (VDF); diabetes, jaundice, hepatitis, and worms (RAR). It is also used in poultices for external cuts and sores (AED).

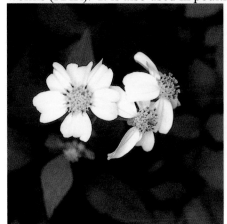

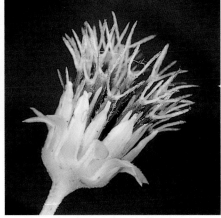

Fig. 26   The distinctive daisy-like flowers of Spanish needles.

Fig. 27   The two-pronged animal-dispersed seeds of Spanish needles.

Angel's Trumpet
Toé

Latin Name: ***Brugmansia suaveolens*** **(H.&B. ex Willd.) Berchtold**
Solanaceae: Nightshade or Potato Family   & Presl

Description: Angel's trumpet is a herbaceous cultivated plant which
sometimes reaches the size of a large shrub (3-4 meters). The thin leaves are
alternate in arrangement, cordate to lanceolate in shape, and have entire
margins. They may range in size from 8-15cm long by 3-5cm wide. A
definite petiole is present, ranging from 3-7cm long in smaller leaves to 10-
12cm long in larger ones. Very small leaves may be present on the stem above
where the petiole attaches, or opposite a much larger leaf. The large pendent
flowers are funnelform and white or white at the base turning pink towards the
apex, although buds may be yellowish. The flowers are showy and large (20-
25cm), and although borne singly from the leaf axils, often occur in large
numbers. Spent blossoms can often be found at the base of the plant, while
the large (10-15cm) green 'pods'(= calyx) from which they emerge are
retained and visible at the base of healthy blossoms.

Uses: The leaves of angel's trumpet are used to treat various aches and
pains, and are sometimes mixed with the seeds by some Indian groups and
used as a narcotic (SAR). An infusion is used as a calmant and to relieve
tension and anxiety (AED). The leaves are one of the additives used in the
preparation of the hallucinogenic drink *ayahuasca* or *yagé*, as well as in the
formulation of the arrow-poison curare (see Discussion, page 8)(AMP).

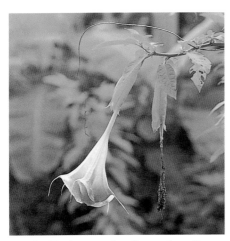

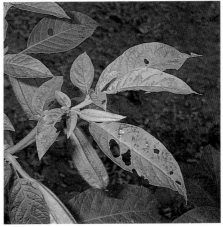

Fig. 33   The large pendent flower of angel's
trumpet.

Fig. 34   Leaves and buds of the angel's
trumpet.

Fever Tree
Chiric Sanango

Latin Name: *Brunfelsia grandiflora* D. Don
Solanaceae: Nightshade or Potato Family

Description: This species grows wild as a small tree throughout tropical South America, while the subspecies *schultesii* is cultivated (SAR). The leaves are somewhat thickened, simple, entire, and alternate in arrangement. They are oval-shaped with a definite drip-tip, range from 10-13cm long by 3-5cm wide, and are borne on a very short (1cm) petiole. The secondary veins originating from the midrib are distinctive if not prominent. Their pattern can be described as alternate loops, never reaching the leaf edge, but rather doubling back on the next vein. The flowers are 2-3cm in diameter, lavender, and have a long (3-6cm) narrow tubular base. They emerge in protruding rather than rounded buds. The fruits are round, green, smooth and about 2-4cm in diameter. They occur in small clusters on upright stalks of 2-4cm length.

Uses: This tree is commonly used in the treatment of fever throughout the northwest region of the Amazon Basin, probably because one of the effects of taking it is to experience chills. Some Indian groups use it by itself as a hallucinogen, but it has gained more widespread indigenous use as an additive in the preparation of *ayahuasca* (see Discussion, page 8). Fever tree is taken in the form of a brew from the leaves or bark, and as a root infusion. Some of the ailments it has been used to cure are yellow fever, syphilis, rheumatism, arthritis, and snakebite (SAR). It is also an additive in some forms of curare.

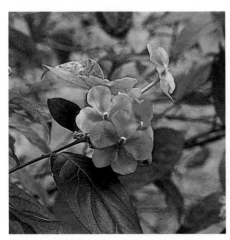

Fig. 35   A cluster of flowers of the fever tree (*Brunfelsia grandiflora*).

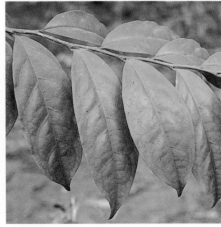

Fig. 36   Leaves of the fever tree (*Brunfelsia grandiflora*).

Pride of Barbados
Angel Sisa

Latin Name: *Caesalpinia pulcherrima* (L.) Sw.
Caesalpiniaceae: Caesalpinia Family

Description: This species is a cultivated shrub or small tree. The leaves
are alternate and even bipinnately compound with typically 14-18 pinnae.
Each pinna has approximately 18-22 leaflets which are oblong-elliptic in
shape. The leaves are 30-40cm long by 10-15cm wide. The inflorescence
occurs in a cluster (= panicle) in pyramidal formation. Most of the showy
flowers are orange-red with yellow fringes, although some may be nearly all
yellow. They are approximately 2-3cm in diameter, and have long (6-7cm)
red stamens that protrude from the front of the blossom. The fruit is a flat
pod (= legume) that grows up to 12cm in length. There are usually some
thorns present along the stem.

Uses: This plant is mostly used as an ornamental due to the bright colorful
flowers. An extract of the leaves is used as a strong laxative and also to stun
fish (SOU). The bark is used in preparations to reduce fevers. It also func-
tions to induce abortions (AED). The flowers can also be used as a laxative,
as well as in treatments to combat fever (AED).

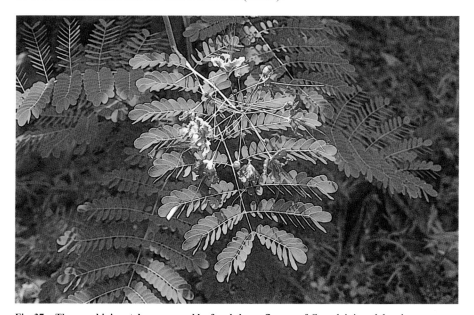

Fig. 37   The even bipinnately compound leaf and showy flowers of *Caesalpinia pulcherrima*.

Firewood Tree
Capirona

Latin Name: *Calycophyllum* **spp.**
Capirona **spp.**
Rubiaceae: Madder or Coffee Family

Description: The Spanish name *capirona* is given to at least three species in the genus *Calycophyllum* (*C. spruceanum*, *C. acreanum*, and *C. obovatum*)(AED), as well as to two species in the genus *Capirona* itself (AHG). The main identifying feature of all of these trees is their thin, papery, smooth, peeling bark. In some species it has a distinctly reddish color to it, while in others the trunk appears green-grey.

Uses: As the English common name implies, *capirona* is often used as a wood for cooking fires, and in the manufacture of charcoal. Stacks of *capirona* cord wood drying in the sun are a common sight in the Upper Amazon. *C. spruceanum* is used as a bark extract by some natives to treat diabetes (RVM). The powdered bark of the same species is used to treat fungal infections (SAR).

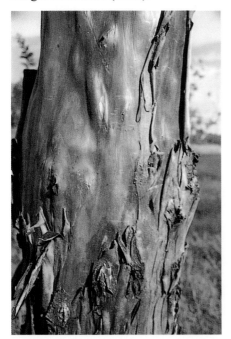 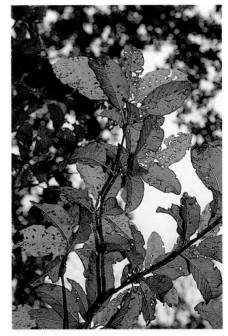

Fig. 38   The trunk and bark of a *capirona* tree.   Fig. 39   The branch and leaves of a *capirona* tree.

Papaya
Papaya

Latin Name: *Carica papaya* L.
Caricaceae: Papaya Family

Description: Papaya is native to the Neotropics, but is now cultivated throughout the tropics worldwide. It is a large, upright perennial herb that can sometimes reach a height of eight meters with a trunk 10-15cm in diameter. It has large, deeply-lobed, simple succulent leaves that may be 30-40cm wide. Leaves are borne on long (50-80cm) petioles and usually grow in a whorl around the entire stem, but clustered at the top. They exude a white milky latex when torn or broken off. Flowering plants produce clusters of white blossoms with yellow centers. The flowers have five petals, a long tubular calyx, and are about 2cm in diameter. The fruit of papaya is generally pear-shaped, green, and ranges from 1-10kg in weight. The fruits are thick-skinned and have an orange or yellow flesh inside and dozens of round black seeds.

Uses: Papayas are rich in Vitamin C and are easily digested. They are eaten raw when ripe, cooked when immature, and are also blended into a thick juice. Various Indian groups employ papaya as a vermifuge, using either the latex or the seeds. The unripe fruit can be grated and eaten with aspirin to induce an abortion (SAR). Immature papayas are also eaten to initiate menstruation and to induce labor, while the sap is applied topically to treat wounds and infections (MC). Papaya enzymes have been used in meat tender-izers and to dissolve tissue in the treatment of herniated discs (AED).

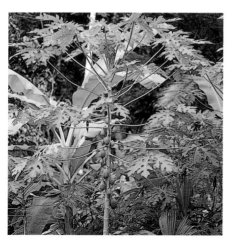

Fig. 40   Crown of papaya tree. Note the deeply lobed palmate leaves and fruits on the trunk.

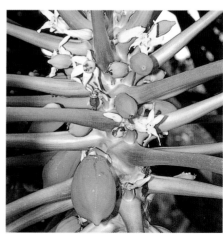

Fig. 41   Papaya flowers and developing fruits on the top of the trunk amongst the petioles.

Panama Hat 'Palm'
Bombonaje

Latin Name: *Carludovica palmata* R. & P.
Cyclanthaceae: Cyclanth Family

Description: The Panama hat 'palm' produces leaf blades that are pleated or fan-shaped from petioles that may reach a length of 3.5 meters. The leaves (petiole + blade) emerge from near ground level and usually occur in a dense compact cluster. The whitish staminate and pistillate flowers occur on a fleshy, almost cylindrical spike (= spadix). This spike is green when the fruits are immature and may be 20-30cm long and 4-6cm in diameter. The spike is borne on a stalk that may be 40-60cm long. The fruits are berries that turn bright orange at maturity and fall away from the spike. Although this plant has palm-like foliage, it is not a palm.

Uses: Medicinally, the plant roots are used to relieve the soreness of bruises (AED) and for relief of stingray stings (RAR). The petioles can be separated into thin segments and used to make baskets, fans, blowgun darts, and most famous, Panama hats (AED). The latter is a misnomer given that such hats are made in Ecuador. Some indigenous Indian groups eat the buds (AED).

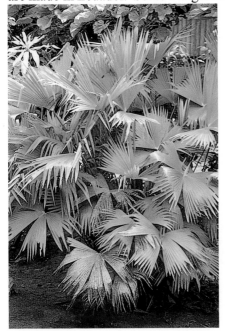

Fig. 42   The dense, fan-like leaves of the Panama hat 'palm'.

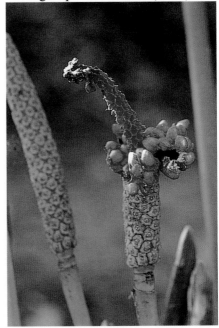

Fig. 43   The mature fruit spike of the Panama hat 'palm'.

Kapok
Lupuna, Ceiba

Latin Name: *Ceiba pentandra* **(L.) Gaertn.**
Bombacaceae: Balsa Family

Description: The kapok is one of the largest trees found in the rainforest and is characterized by large buttress roots at the base and a giant spreading crown at the top. These emergent trees often grew along the rivers which made them highly visible and easily accessible targets for lumbering operations. The small flowers occur in massive numbers for a single night, attracting hundreds of pollinating bats. The fruits are large 20-25cm long, red elliptical, woody capsules. Within the fruits, the seeds are embedded in a cottony, floss-like material (kapok) that provides for their aerial dispersal. Trees loaded with these hanging red fruits are often seen from the rivers, while the kapok material itself is frequently evident within the forest at times when it has drifted down onto the foliage from the ripe capsules above.

Uses: Kapok has been used by the timber industry for decades as a source of lumber for plywood production. As a result of over exploitation, it is now scarce in many places where it was once abundant. The wooly kapok floss was once used to stuff pillows, mattresses, and life preservers. Indigenous Indians use this 'silk' as fletching for their blowgun darts, often keeping a supply in a woven fiber bag or a gourd. Brews made from the branches have been used both as an emetic and a diuretic (VDF). The bark of kapok has been used in baths as a treatment to alleviate fever (AED).

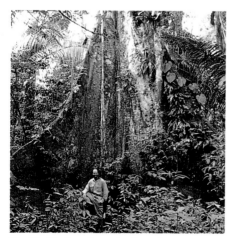

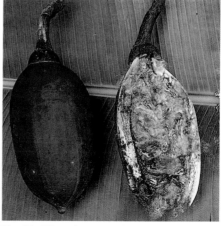

Fig. 44 The kapok tree has large buttress roots at its base as shown here with author (JLC).

Fig. 45 The red capsular fruit of the kapok tree contains a cottony material (kapok) inside.

Wormseed
Paico

Latin Name: *Chenopodium ambrosioides* L.
Chenopodiaceae: Goosefoot Family

Description: Wormseed is a weedy looking herb that grows to a meter in height. This plant is very aromatic and found mainly in the dry areas of the Andes Mountains, as well as in various disturbed areas. The leaves are simple and alternate with large distinct teeth along the margin. The slender leaves are generally lanceolate in shape, measuring 4-5cm long by .5-1cm wide. They narrow towards the base but do not appear to have distinct petioles. The flowers are very small, greenish-colored, and are borne in clusters along a single stalk or axis (= spike). Small flower spikes with whorls of tiny leaves are common in the leaf axils. The small round green fruits are only several millimeters in diameter.

Uses: This plant is an effective treatment for getting rid of intestinal worms in young children (AMP). It is given as a warm tea of leaves and seeds to women about to have babies in order to accelerate delivery (AMP). Due to the aromatic nature of the plant, one Indian tribe uses it as a perfume (SAR). The AED lists numerous medical problems for which wormseed is used including tuberculosis, gout, hemorrhoids, cholera, tumors, fever, flu, and stomachache. In Mexico, wormseed is sometimes used as a spice. A plant in the same genus (*Chenopodium quinoa*) produces a nutritious grain (quinoa) that has been cultivated at higher altitudes in the Andes since Incan times.

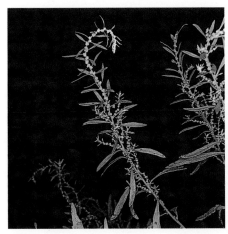
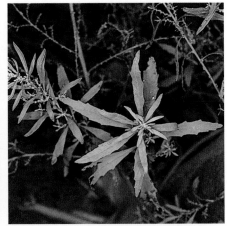

Fig. 46 Wormseed showing leaves and flower or fruit spikes.

Fig. 47 The whorled, toothed leaves of wormseed.

Curare
Curaré

Latin Name: *Chondrodendron tomentosum* **R. & P.**
Menispermaceae: Moonseed Family

Description: This plant grows to be a large canopy liana that may get as thick as 10cm in diameter at its base. It has alternate, simple, entire cordate leaves. The leaves may be 10-20cm long and almost the same wide with a 5-15cm long petiole (TBC). The leaves are smooth above and hairy white below, with veins radiating palmately from the leaf base. The inflorescences consist of separate clusters of male and female flowers, each of which is small (1-2mm), greenish-white, and inconspicuous. The fleshy fruits are oval-oblong, approximately 1-2mm long, and narrow at the base (TBC).

Uses: Various Indian tribes throughout the Amazon Basin use an extract of this plant as the main ingredient in preparing curare, a potent jungle poison (see Discussion, page 8). The roots and stem of this plant are cooked, along with the bark and seeds of *Strychnos* spp. (page 121) and other botanical additives, as well as various venemous frogs and insects. Amazonian Indians coat the tips of their blowgun darts with the curare. When the dart penetrates the flesh of an animal that is 'shot' during hunting, alkaloids in the poison take affect to render the animal helpless and easily captured. Other uses of this plant by Amazonian natives include as a diuretic and to treat fever (SAR). It is also used to alleviate swelling and as a remedy for kidney stones (RAR).

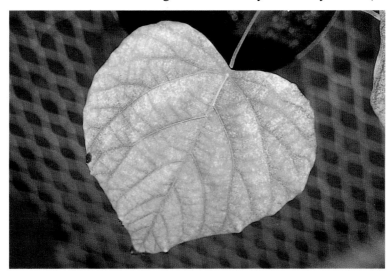

Fig. 48 Leaf of a young *Chondrodendron tomentosum* plant. (Photo by Boyce Tankersley)

Caimito

Caimito

Latin Name: *Chrysophyllum cainito* L.
Sapotaceae: Sapodilla Family

Description: Caimito is a medium-sized tree (15-25m) with a scaly grayish outer bark that reveals a light brown color beneath. The trunks are angular rather than round in cross-section. The ovate leaves are simple, alternate, and entire, terminating in a small but distinctive point. Mature leaves range from 10-12cm in length by 5-6cm in width and are borne on a short (1-2cm) twisted woody petiole. The secondary veins are parallel, closely-spaced, and almost perpendicular to the midvein. Mature leaves are a shiny dark green on their upper surfaces and covered with satiny copper-red brown colored hairs on the under surfaces. This brown satiny covering extends down the midrib and along the branches. New leaves emerge folded in half with only the brown underside showing which contrasts greatly with dark green mature leaves. Caimito produces many small, beige-colored flowers that develop into rounded fruits approximately 5-10cm in diameter. The fruits are green while young but mature to purple. Caimito is sometimes called star fruit, but should not be confused with *Averrhoa carambola* (page 20) or *Clusia rosea* (page 39). Caimito produces a milky latex characteristic of the sapodilla family.

Uses: Caimito has edible fruits and is found cultivated in tropical lowland areas of Central and northern South America. Native Indians use the latex as a treatment for infected gums as well as for fungal crotch infections (SAR). It has also been used to treat open sores (RAR).

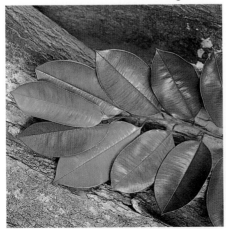

Fig. 49   The shiny dark green upper surface of caimito leaves.

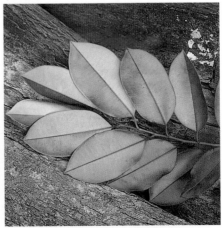

Fig. 50   The satiny coppery-brown under surface of caimito leaves.

38

Toad Vine
Sapo Huasca

Latin Name: *Cissus sicyoides* L.
Vitaceae: Grape Family

Description: Toad vine is an understory liana that is found in much of South America, Central America, and even the southern United States. It has alternate leaves, often with tendrils occurring opposite to them. The simple leaves are narrowly ovate to obovate, coming to a point at the tip. The margins have distinct teeth at regular intervals and the leaves are petiolate. Several veins radiate palmately from the base, while lateral veins extend out from the midrib to the teeth at the leaf margin. Inflorescences are clusters of small (3mm or less) flowers whose color depends on the available light. In shaded areas the blossoms are greenish white to yellow, while in open sunny areas they are red. The ovoid fruits are 5-6mm long and turn from green to red to black as they develop. (TBC)

Uses: Toad vine is used in a manner similar to *Kalanchoe pinnata* (page 69). The leaves, stems, and flowers are mixed and crushed to form a thick material which is applied fresh directly to tumors. It is believed to alleviate the heat, pain, and inflammation, eventually removing the tumor (AMP). This is one of the most commonly employed pain relievers (AED). In various applications it has been used to treat flu (RAR), as a tea for anemia (BDS), and as a poultice on sprains (NIC). The English and Spanish names come from the resemblance of the compound leaves of related species to a frogs foot.

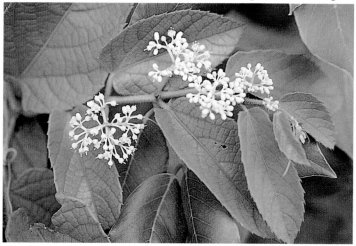

Fig. 51   The leaves and flowers of toad vine.   (Photo by Walter Judd)

Clusia
Renaquilla

Latin Name: *Clusia rosea* Jacq.
Clusiaceae: Clusia Family

Description: *Clusia* spp. are hemiepiphytic shrubs and trees. This species
should not be confused with the edible star fruit or carambola (*Averrhoa
carambola*)(page 20), which is grown worldwide. The thick, succulent leaves
are simple and opposite, a dark shiny green above and light green below. The
leaves are generally ovate to obovate in form and have entire margins. They
range from 15-40cm long by 10-20cm wide. A yellow midvein is usually
visible, while parallel secondary veins running almost perpendicular to it are
indistinct. The leaves are borne on substantial petioles that are 3-5cm in
length. The fruit is a capsule which is star-shaped when open.

Uses: The bark of larger trees produces a yellowish resin when cut or
injured. When mixed with water that is then boiled and taken orally, it is said
to have properties that promote the healing of internal fractures, including
injuries to the ribs and back (AMP). The bark is also used for rheumatism
(AED). The large thick leaves were once used for written messages (RVM).

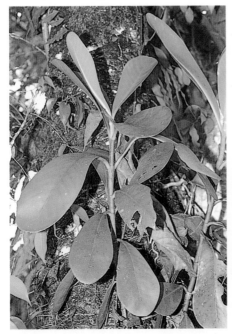
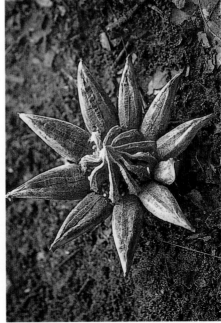

Fig. 52   A young star fruit tree (*Clusia rosea*).   Fig. 53   Star-like fruit of *Clusia rosea*.

Coffee
Café

Latin Name: *Coffea* **spp.**
Rubiaceae: Madder or Coffee Family

Description: Coffee is a cultivated shrub with dense foliage and a bushy appearance. Slender branches project off a small central trunk and bear simple opposite leaves with wavy, entire margins. The leaves are usually shiny, 10-12cm long by 3-4cm wide, and terminate in an extended point or drip-tip. The clusters of small white flowers arise in the upper angle between the leaf and the stem (= axillary). Many fruits (= berries) are produced in clusters of 15-25 between the opposite pairs of leaves. The immature berries are green, but turn red as they ripen and grow to a size of about 1-2cm.

Uses: Coffee is consumed the world over as a beverage brewed from the ground seed or 'bean' of the coffee plant. It is also used as a flavoring agent. Earliest uses involved using the fruits to make a juice, which could also be fermented and made into a wine. Indigenous Africans chewed both the leaves and the beans as a stimulant, similar to the use of coca by the montane Indians of the Andes in South America. In Brazil, a brew is made from both the leaves and the beans and drunk to accelerate labor (BDS). It is also used in the treatment of pulmonary problems, and against the flu (RAR).

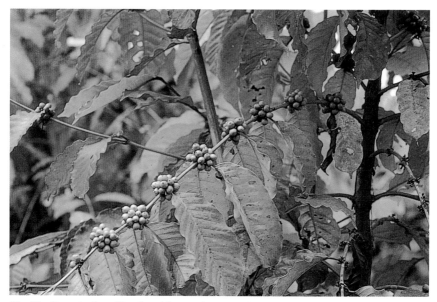

Fig. 54   **Branch of a coffee plant (*C. canephora*) heavily laden with immature 'beans'.**

Two main types of coffee are grown commercially, both of which originated in Africa. Arabica coffee (*Coffea arabica*) is a montane species grown throughout the tropics at elevations ranging from roughly 1,000-2,000 meters. It originated on the slopes of the mountainous tropical forests of Ethiopia. It is generally considered to produce the best coffee in terms of flavor and quality. Robusta coffee (*Coffea canephora*) is a lowland species that originated in the Congo River Basin. Brazil is one of the major producers of this coffee, which grows better in the conditions that prevail in the humid tropics. (SWPT)

Arabs were the first to originally cultivate coffee as a crop and roast the 'beans'. Coffee consumption became popular in Europe in the late 1600's. Coffee cultivation was introduced into the New World in the early 1700's by the Dutch in Dutch Guiana and by the French on the island of Martinique. Subsequent introductions derived from these plantings were made throughout Latin America and the Caribbean. Coffee is the developing world's largest legal agricultural export commodity. (SWPT)

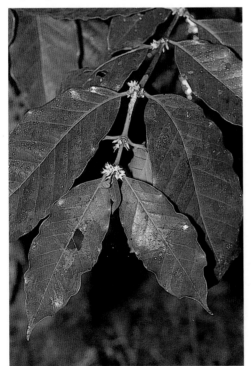

Fig. 55   Coffee flowers and leaves (*C. arabica*).

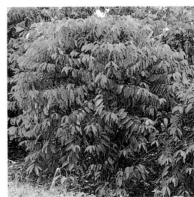

Fig. 56   A coffee bush about two meters tall.

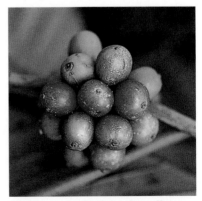

Fig. 57   A cluster of ripening coffee 'beans'.

Pineapple Ginger
Cañagre

Latin Name: *Costus lasius* Loes.
Costaceae: Costus Family

Description: This is a tall perennial herb that occurs in clusters 2-3m high. Large fleshy entire leaves with clasping sheaths are arranged spirally around the 2-3cm diameter stem. The leaves are lanceolate to ovate, pointed, and range in size from 12-30cm long by 5-10cm wide. The midvein has many long nearly parallel veins that diverge from it. The flowers emerge from a fleshy green cone composed of whorls of overlapping bracts with outwardly projecting tips that resemble the green foliage found on top of a pineapple fruit. Cones are from 15-25cm long and about 8-12cm wide, located at the top of stems that are less than a meter in height and below where the plant foliage begins. Emerging flower buds are white-pink, while the blossom itself is pink at the base and red and yellow at the opening. They are broadly tubular and about 7-10cm long by 2-3cm in diameter.

Uses: The leaves of this cañagre have the recorded use of staunching the flow of blood from arrow wounds (GMJ).

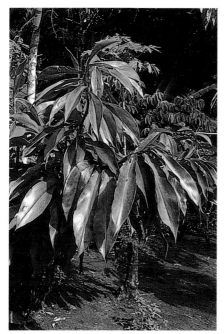

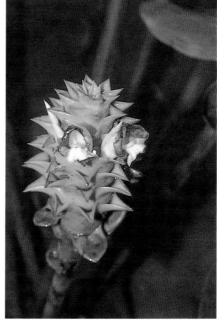

Fig. 58   The leaves of *Costus lasius*.

Fig. 59   Flowers and 'cone' of *Costus lasius*.

Candlestick Ginger
Cañagre

Latin Name: *Costus scaber* R. & P.
Costaceae: Costus Family

Description: This plant is a large perennial herb that usually occurs in clusters 2-3m high. The large fleshy entire leaves have clasping sheathes and are arranged spirally around the 2-3cm diameter stem. The leaves are ovate to lanceolate, pointed, and range from 12-30cm long by 5-10cm wide. Many secondary veins run nearly parallel to the midvein. The squarishly tubular yellow-orange flowers are about 2cm wide by 4-5cm long and project from an orange-red cone of tightly overlapping scales (= bracts), located at the top of the stem. The cone may be 8-20cm long and usually has one or two blossoms.

Uses: Young plants (.5m or less) are crushed and the juice extracted for treatment of internal fever and bronchitis (AMP). A decoction from the root is used to treat stomachaches and snakebites (AED). The juice of crushed flowers and leaves is taken orally by some as a treatment for worms, although vaginal infections are treated by one Indian group by using a douche made of the flowers (AED). Other tribes use it for liver ailments (SOU).

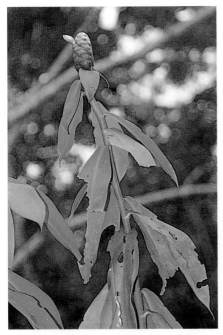
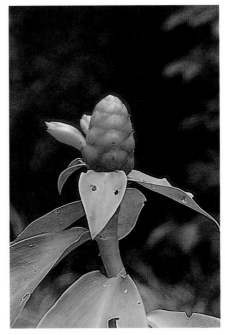

Fig. 60   Stem and leaves of *Costus scaber*.   **Fig. 61   Flower and 'cone' of *Costus scaber*.**

Milk Tree
Leche Caspi

Latin Name: *Couma macrocarpa* **Barb.**
Apocynaceae: Dogbane Family

Description: This species is a large tree with a copious milky latex for which it is named (both Spanish and English). The foliage is distinctive with large broad stiff leathery whorled leaves that occur in threes at each of the nodes. This symmetry of threes gives milk tree a certain recognizable growth form. The leaves are simple, entire, oval-shaped and pointed at the apex. Mature leaves range from 20-40cm long by 10-25cm wide. There is a distinctive yellow midvein, with parallel secondary veins that are nearly perpendicular to the midvein at the leaf base, but increasing in the angle of intersection towards the tip. The short (2-3cm) woody brown petiole is slightly expanded at its base. Clusters of small (1-2cm) flowers are borne on the ends of stalks that also occur in threes at the nodes. The round fruits are 2-4cm in diameter.

Uses: Both the fruits and the latex of the milk tree are edible. This species has been used commercially both to supply a latex substitute for chewing gum (page 78) and as an additive to rubber (SAR). Several Indian groups in the Peruvian Amazon chew dried milk tree leaves when *coca* leaves (page 52) are not available (SAR). The latex is used to treat amoebic dysentery, as well as skin irritations (RVM). In some areas the latex is used to heal the umbilical scar of newborns, while in others it is taken as a purgative (SAR). One tribe uses the ground powdered bark of the tree as an antiseptic (VDF).

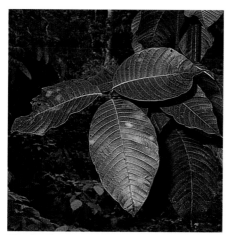

Fig. 62   The three- whorled simple leaves of the milk tree.

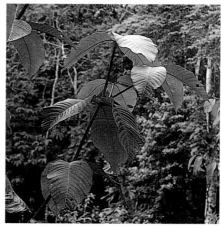

Fig. 63   The 'symmetry of threes' gives the milk tree a distinctive growth form.

Calabash
Huingo

Latin Name: *Crescentia cujete* L.
Bignoniaceae: Trumpet Vine or Catalpa Family

Description: The calabash tree is a small (3-5 meters) tree that is native to tropical America. The simple, entire leaves are clustered together in whorl-like bunches or fascicles. Leaves are oblanceolate, being wide at the tip which ends in a short point, and becoming very narrow at the base. Larger leaves may be 20-25cm long by 8-10cm wide at their widest point. Flowers are produced directly from the branches and the trunk (= cauliflory), subsequently developing into the fruit for which the tree is named. The pale night-blooming flowers are tinged with green and pink, and emerge from bright green buds on small stalks. The flowers are about 4-6cm long by 4-6cm in diameter. The large (20-40cm) round fruit is bright green and may weigh up to 10kg. It is hard-shelled and contains seeds embedded in a fleshy pulp. The overall size, shape, and growth habit of the calabash tree is remindful of an apple tree.

Uses: The most widespread use of the calabash tree is for making water gourds or containers from the hollowed out fruits. The hard-shelled fruits are also used to make maracas, and serve as a medium for carvings and etchings that are sold to tourists. In certain areas, natives chew the leaves of this tree to relieve toothaches (SAR). Other medicinal uses of this species include the preparation of treatments for asthma, diarrhea and intestinal problems, hernias and sprains, and as an abortive and a purgative (AED).

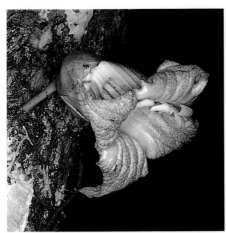

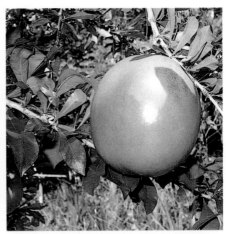

Fig. 64 Night-blooming flower of the calabash tree growing directly from a trunk.

Fig. 65 A calabash, the fruit of the calabash tree.

Dragon's Blood
Sangre del Grado

Latin Name: *Croton lechleri* Muell.-Arg.
Euphorbiaceae: Spurge Family

Description: This species is a medium-sized tree, fairly open in growth habit and with the leaves tending to be clustered towards the ends of the branches. Dragon's blood is so named because the bark when cut exudes a reddish to orange latex. The simple, alternate, entire leaves are heart-shaped (= cordate) and terminate in a long narrow drip-tip. Leaves range in size from approximately 15-30cm long by 15-30cm wide, and are borne on long petioles that range from 15-30cm in length. There are three main veins that radiate palmately from the leaf base, as well as 6-8 obvious parallel secondary veins that diverge diagonally from the midvein. The larger veins and petiole are covered with what appears to be tiny bumps or hairs (= trichomes) that rub off. The smaller veins have a 'dotted' appearance. The small flowers are borne on a tall slender upright spike from 30-50cm long. The fruits are three-parted capsules.

Uses: Many species of *Croton* are used by indigenous people as a purgative, while the sap from some forms the main constituent of certain varnishes (SAR). The red resin of dragon's blood is taken orally in hot water to hasten internal healing following an abortion (AMP). The sap is also used to staunch the flow of blood and heal wounds (NIC). It is used as a vaginal douche subsequent to childbirth (AED), and to treat tuberculosis and bone cancer (AMP). Two drugs derived from this plant are currently in clinical trials.

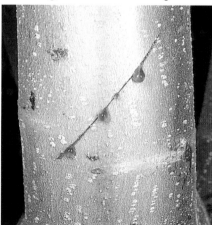

Fig. 66   Dragon's blood exudes a red latex if cut.

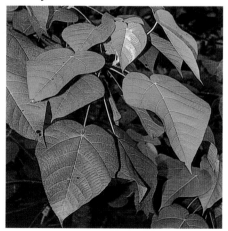

Fig. 67   Distinctive foliage of dragon's blood.

Turmeric
Guisador

Latin Name: *Curcuma longa* L.
Zingiberaceae: Ginger Family

Description: Turmeric is a rhizomatous herb that is native to the Orient, but also cultivated in the Amazon Basin region. This member of the ginger family has alternate, two-ranked, entire leaves with the parallel venation that is characteristic of monocotyledonous plants. The bases of the leaves form sheathes around the stems. The inflorescence is a dense spike of perfect flowers, each of which is surrounded by a large bract. The flowers are irregular, having three sepals and three petals. Some of the stamens resemble petals (= petaloid). The fruit is a capsule. Turmeric produces large, thickened orange underground stems (= rhizomes).

Uses: The underground rhizomes of this plant are dried and ground into a powder that is also called turmeric and used as a spice, often incorporated into curry powder (SAO). This powder is also used as a yellow dye for bark cloth and woven materials in Papua New Guinea, Asia, and the Amazon region (AL, SAR). Some Indian groups wear the aromatic leaves as perfume by wrapping them around their arms (SAR). The juice from crushed rhizomes mixed with water is taken orally to treat hepatitis (AED). The crushed rhizomes are also mixed with other plants such as *Siparuna guianensis* (page 116) and other ingredients when used as a poultice to relieve bruises (AED). Several antiinflammatory compounds have been found in the rhizomes (AED).

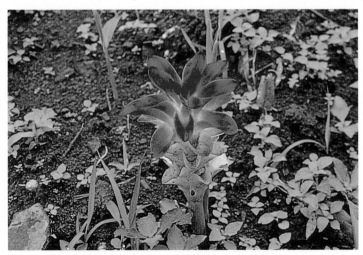

Fig. 68   Inflorescence of turmeric.   (Photo by Alan Meerow)

Lemon Grass
Hierba Luisa

Latin Name: *Cymbopogon citratus* (DC.) Stapf.
Poaceae: Grass Family

Description: Lemon grass is an introduced plant that is grown as a cultivated herb in the Amazon region. It has long (30-60cm), narrow (1-3cm), leaves that sheath the stem at their base. The blades grow grouped together, several to a fascicle. They have parallel venation which is indistinct. The leaf blades are rough and somewhat saw-like to touch. A typical clump of lemon grass is 90-120cm in diameter. The leaves are highly aromatic (due to oils present) and when bruised or crushed, give off the odor of lemons.

Uses: Lemon grass is cultivated and used in various culinary dishes as an herb. An extract of the leaves is used in making carbonated drinks, and also as a digestive aid (AED). Amazonian Indians use the leaves in preparations to treat fever, headache, influenza, and stomachache (SAR). The roots are squeezed and the extract used to control menstrual problems (AED), and to relieve backaches and muscle spasms. Essential oils are extracted and used commercially in soaps and perfumes. Certain preparations of lemon grass are also used by some indigenous groups as a contraceptive (VDF).

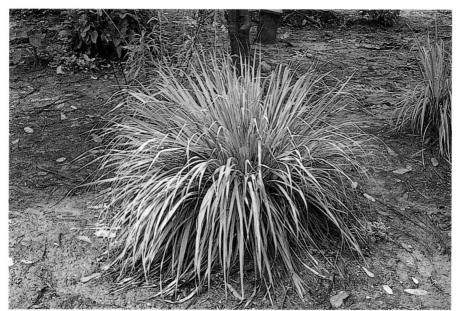

Fig. 69   A typical clump of lemon grass (*Cymbopogon citratus*).

Fer-de-lance Plant
Jergón Sacha

Latin Name: ***Dracontium loretense*** **Krause**
Araceae: Arum Family

Description: This plant is a terrestrial herb that grows as a forest under-story plant. It puts forth a single, large, highly dissected leaf borne on a long, straight, erect fleshy petiole which may range from 50-200cm in height. It can reach a diameter of several centimeters, and has a brown/green/gray mottled pattern that is reminiscent of that found on some snakes (accounting for the name). The plane of the leaf is parallel to the ground, making the plant look like a miniature tree. The sole leaf is so highly dissected that it appears to be several asymmetrical pinnately compound leaves arranged in a whorl. The inflorescence is 15-25cm long, borne on a separate long stalk, and has a spike of numerous white flowers (= spadix) nearly totally surrounded by an upcurv-ing hoodlike structure (= spathe) which is greenish outside and purplish inside.

Uses: A drink made from the large, bulbous root cut into pieces and boiled in water is used for the immediate treatment of snakebite (AMP). The tuber may also be heated and applied directly to the wound itself (JAD).

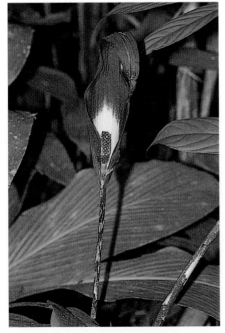

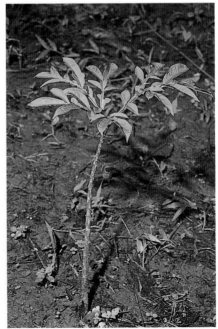

Fig. 70   The fer-de-lance plant inflorescence usually grows at the same height as the leaf.

Fig. 71   The highly dissected leaf and long upright petiole of the fer-de-lance plant.

Wild Coriander
Sacha Culantro

Latin Name: *Eryngium foetidum* L.
Apiaceae: Carrot Family

Description: Wild coriander is a common weed of the lowland tropics often found in disturbed areas. It grows as a perennial herb, reaching 60cm. The basal, ground-level leaves are linear, distinctly and regularly serrate, and about 10-15cm long by 3-5cm wide. The small upper leaves are variable in shape, but are arranged in rosettes that give them a star-like appearance. The most common leaf forms are either slender and lanceolate, pointed at the tip, and with several very small teeth produced into fine points along the otherwise entire margin; or leaves twice as wide with a 3-pointed tip and larger more distinctive teeth along the edges. The upper leaves observed were 2-3cm long by 1-2cm wide. Clusters of tiny (1-2mm) flowers are borne in small green cylindrical heads approximately 5-10mm high by 5mm in diameter. They are found at the ends of branches with 5-6 leaf-like bracts in a rosette at their base. If any part of the plant is crushed, it produces a distinctive pungent odor.

Uses: Wild coriander is cultivated by many inhabitants throughout the New World tropics where it is used as a condiment to add a distinctive flavor to otherwise non-descript dishes. The taste is pleasing to some, but overpowering to others. A brew made from the plant is used in Central America to treat indigestion, diarrhea, and vomiting in young children (AAB). It is also used to dispel flatulence (AAB).

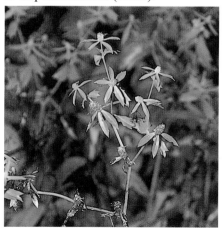

Fig. 72   Growth form of wild coriander.

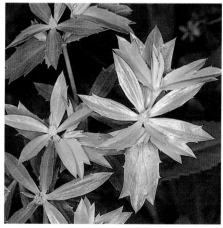

Fig. 73   Flower heads and upper leaves of wild coriander.

Swamp Immortelle
Amasisa

Latin Name: *Erythrina fusca* **Lour.**
Fabaceae: Pea or Bean Family

Description: Swamp immortelle is a medium-sized tree reaching a height of 15-20m, bearing short prickles on the branches. The alternate, compound leaves are trifoliate, with the central or terminal leaflet slightly larger than the lateral ones. The terminal leaflet is approximately 10-15cm long by 8-10cm wide. All leaflets have a visible yellow midvein that is most obvious in the basal half. The petiole is 10-15cm long and rounded and slightly swollen at its base. A pair of bump-like glands are present at the base of each leaflet and at the apex of the petiole. These glands are very noticeable on the uncurled, coppery-colored new leaves. The flowers are large, orange, and showy, occurring in pendent clusters on thick stalks (= pedicels). The long, slender bean-like fruits are roughly 20cm long by 2cm wide, pointed at the tip, and are covered with a dense brown layer of hair (TBC).

Uses: This tree is cultivated in some areas, and because it roots easily and has showy flowers has been used in the establishment of 'living fences'(SAR). In some areas they are also planted to add nitrogen to the soil (AED). Medicinally, bark preparations of swamp immortelle have been used to treat skin and fungal infections, as well as to clean out infected wounds (AED). The bark is used with water to treat inflamed kidneys (AMP). Some indigenous groups use a root preparation as a treatment for the fevers with malaria (AED). A bark water bath is used for severe headaches (AMP).

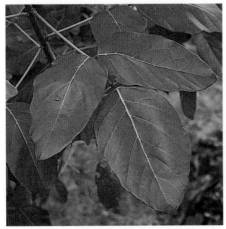
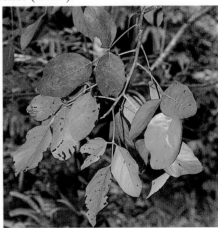

Fig. 74   The trifoliate compound leaf of swamp immortelle.

Fig. 75   Foliage of swamp immortelle.

Coca, Cocaine Bush
Coca

Latin Name: *Erythroxylon coca* **Lamarck var.** *ipadu* **Plowman**
Erythroxylaceae: Cocaine Family

Description: This plant is one of several species from which cocaine is derived, and may also be listed with the genus spelled *Erythroxylum*. Coca plants are understory shrubs with simple, entire, alternate leaves. The leaves are smooth, oval-shaped, and approximately 5-8cm long, borne on short petioles. The inconspicuous flowers are small and white and are found singly or in small clusters along the branches or in the leaf axils. The red, berry-like, elliptical fruits contain a single seed and are borne on a short stalk.

Uses: The coca plant, like the vine *ayahuasca* or *yagé* (*Banisteriopsis caapi*, page 21), has a long history of use by indigenous peoples. While cocaine today bears the stigma of a recreational drug, coca leaves have been chewed by Andean Indians of South America in a tradition that dates back thousands of years. This has been confirmed by various archaeological artifacts discovered. The coca leaves contain alkaloids that have the effect of increasing energy, decreasing hunger, and that may result in feelings of euphoria. Coca leaves are prepared as a chew or in powder form, and are packed in the mouth (DAW). Lime, in the form of ashes of various other plants or from burned rocks, are also added to enhance the flavor and effect. Coca use in the Amazon is traditionally restricted to the males (SAR). It is cultivated widely throughout the Andean countries of South America.

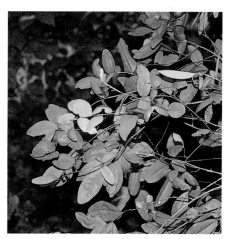

Fig. 76   The foliage of a coca bush
(*Erythroxylon* sp.)

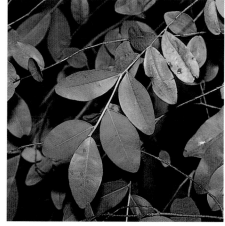

Fig. 77   Leaves of a coca plant
(*Erythroxylon* sp.)

Amazon Lily
Delia

Latin Name: *Eucharis castelnaeana* (Baill.) McBr.
Amaryllidaceae: Amaryllis Family

Description: This species is not a true lily and is the only member of the amaryllis family to occur in lowland tropical forests (AHG). Sometimes listed as *Eucharis amazonica* (SAR), it is easily recognized for both its distinctive flowers and fruits. Amazon lily is a low-growing herb that sprouts from a bulb and can be seen along the forest floor. It usually has two oblong petiolate leaves with parallel venation. A slender, upright, elongated flower stalk (= scape) bearing four or more flowers at its top reaches a height of approximately 20-30cm. The large, showy, white flowers are 4-5cm in diameter and look much like a daffodil blossom in shape. They are somewhat pendent, the basal portion of the flower being a thin, non-rigid tube that is about 5-6cm in length. The fruits are bright orange capsules that reveal black seeds when open. Usually 3-4 capsules are found on erect green stems.

Uses: Amazon lily is grown as an ornamental flower. A tea is also made from the bulb or entire plant and used as an emetic (SAR).

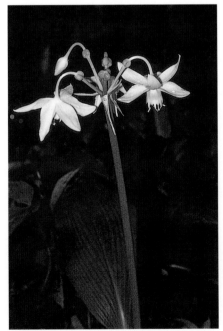 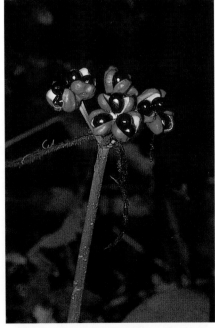

Fig. 78   The daffodil-like flowers of the Amazon lily.

Fig. 79   The distinctive orange capsules and black seeds of the Amazon lily.

Medicinal Fig
Ojé

Latin Name: *Ficus insipida* Willd.
Moraceae: **Fig or Mulberry Family**

Description: Most plants in this genus are strangler figs, but *F. insipida* is a free-living species that can be a large buttressed tree 30-40m in height. The long, broad oval leaves are simple, alternate, and have entire margins that terminate in a short abrupt point. Leaves typically range from 15-30cm long by 8-15cm wide, and are borne on a short (3-5cm) petiole. There is a prominent yellow-green midvein and visible parallel secondary veins, which although originating perpendicular to the midvein curve up towards the tip as they approach the leaf edge. The leaf surface is dark green above and light green below. The rounded to top-shaped fruits are light green in color, about 3-4cm in diameter, and borne singly along the branches on short (1-2cm) stalks. Typical figs are hollow structures with the inside lined with flowers (= synconia) that are pollinated by tiny, species-specific wasps. Broken leaves or cut bark produces a milky white sap.

Uses: This species, as well as many other figs, are reported from multiple sources as having widespread use throughout Amazonia as a purgative against worms and intestinal parasites. The accepted treatment seems to be a mixture of the white latex with sugarcane juice or sugarcane rum (*aguardiente*). The dosage is important since too much of the sap will harm the intestines (AMP). The resin may also burn the skin if it comes in contact with it, although some Indian tribes apply it topically as a treatment for rheumatism (AED).

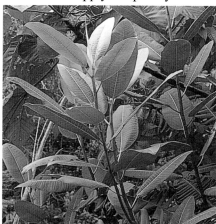

Fig. 80   Growth habit of the medicinal fig
(*Ficus insipida*).

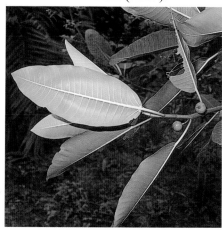

Fig. 81   Leaves and fruits of the medicinal fig
(*Ficus insipida*).

Genipap
Huito

Latin Name: *Genipa americana* L.
Rubiaceae: Madder or Coffee Family

Description: Genipap is a canopy tree that grows to 15-20m tall. It has very large dark green wavy obovate to broadly lanceolate leaves that are clustered at the ends of the branches. The leaves are simple, opposite, have entire margins and a prominent yellow midvein. They range in size from 25-50cm long by 6-20cm wide with a short (1-2cm) petiole. Small clusters of cream to yellow-white flowers are produced. The fruits are round to oval-shaped, brownish at maturity, and approximately 6-8cm in length. They are borne singly on stout brown stalks about 3-4cm long. The sap of the tree is clear at first, but turns blue-black after being exposed to the air.

Uses: The genipap fruit is edible when ripe and is also used to make an alcoholic drink (AED). Juice of the green, immature fruits is used both as a dye for clothing materials and as a face and body paint, oxidizing to a blue-black color after a day or so. The pure juice of ripe fruits is given to children with bronchial problems, while the green fruit juice is a treatment for stomach ulcers (AMP). Ripe fruit is taken with *aguardiente* (by placing the entire fruit in the bottle) to treat arthritis (AMP). Green fruit material is used to extract decaying teeth (AED). A bath of the cooked fruits and seeds is used to wash female genitals when inflamed (AED). In the Caribbean, genipap has been used to treat tumors, anemia, diarrhea, and gonorrhea (DAW).

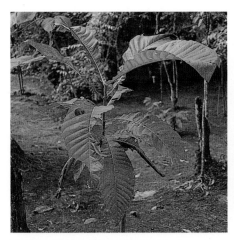

Fig. 82   Leaves of the genipap tree.

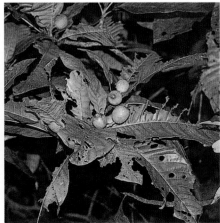

Fig. 83   Mature fruits of the genipap tree.

Cotton
Algodón

Latin Name: *Gossypium* spp.
Malvaceae: Mallow Family

Description: This genus contains about 16 species that are found in the
New World tropics. They are mostly shrubs (some growing to small straggly
trees) in dry habitats and generally reaching heights of 2-5 meters. The plant
typically consists of several slender central trunks or stems that branch. The
simple, alternate leaves are approximately as long as they are wide, but vary
in their overall shape and number of lobes. Most have three or five nearly
equal-sized lobes so that they are similar to the leaves of sassafras and sweet
gum, respectively. They range in size from 7-20cm long by 7-20cm wide.
The large, open flowers are usually beige or yellow with a dark spot inside the
center at the base. Flowers may be 8-10cm in diameter and have large green
leafy triangular structures (bracts) at their base that are fringed with long
narrow teeth. These bracts persist at the base of the large (8-10cm) green
fruit (= boll) which eventually turns brown and splits open to release the seeds
surrounded by fiber (= cotton). The cotton fiber may be white or brown-
colored (*algodón pardo*) depending on the variety.

Uses: Various species of cotton, both native and introduced, are cultivated
in small amounts throughout the Amazon including *G. arboreum, G. hirsutum,
G. barbadense*, and *G. herbaceum*. Medicinal uses include preparations of
the roots as a diuretic and to treat menstrual problems (SAR), the leaves to
hasten childbirth (AED), and the flowers to treat hepatitis (RVM).

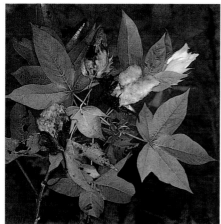

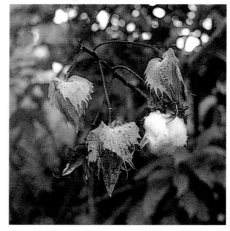

Fig. 84   Leaves, closed green boll (top), open
boll w. fiber, and new blossom of *algodón pardo*.

Fig. 85   Open boll w. cotton fiber and green
bolls w. bracts at base (*Gossypium* sp.).

Wild Mango
Sacha Mango

Latin Name: *Grias neuberthii* Macbr.
Lecythidaceae: Brazil Nut Family

Description: This species is known as wild mango (Spanish and English names), but is unrelated to the true mango (*Mangifera indica*, page 75). It can reach a height of 20-25m, and has a straight trunk that produces few branches. The leaves are simple, alternate, oblanceolate in shape and come to a small point at the tip. They have entire, undulating margins and are arranged in whorls at the ends of the branches and concentrated at the top of the trunk. Leaves range from 30-120cm long by 8-16cm wide and lack petioles, although the blade becomes extremely narrow at the base. The flowers are radially symmetrical with four pale yellow petals that measure 4-6cm across. The flowers develop from round buds in small groups at the ends of stalks (10-20cm long) that project directly from the trunk (= cauliflory) perpendicularly. The ellipsoid fruits are light brown,10-18cm long and 5-10cm wide.

Uses: This tree is grown both as an ornamental and for its edible fruits. The fruits are eaten fresh, roasted, or boiled. In traditional medicine, the fruit pulp is grated and mixed with water to be taken as a purgative (CFNA). The grated seed is used to treat venereal tumors and the fever associated with them (AMP). One group of Amazonian Indians adds the twigs of wild mango to the ingredients in a specific preparation of the dart-poison curare (Discussion, page 8) (SAR). The bark is also used by some groups to promote vomiting, while the seed is used by others as an enema to treat dysentery (SAR).

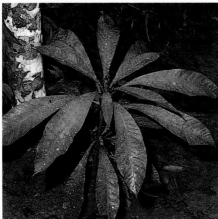 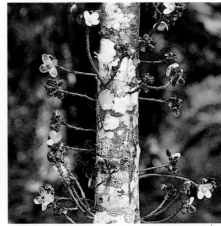

Fig. 86   Cluster of whorled leaves of wild mango tree (*Grias neuberthii*).

Fig. 87   The cauliflorous flowers of wild mango (*Grias neuberthii*).

Heliotrope
Alacransillo

Latin Name: *Heliotropium indicum* L.
Boraginaceae: Forget-Me-Not Family

Description: Heliotrope is an herb that is usually less than a meter in height, becoming straggly when taller. It is a common plant along river banks and sandbars, but is often found in dry areas as well. Heliotrope has simple, entire, alternate, ovate, pointed leaves that have a wrinkled surface and a wavy margin. Most leaves are 5-10cm long by 3-6cm wide with a 2-6cm long petiole. The inflorescence is a narrow cyme 10-30cm long and covered with small lavender flowers curved in a manner that resembles a scorpion's tail (from which the Spanish name is derived: *alacrán* = scorpion). Individual flowers are only 4-5mm in diameter. The developing fruits are smooth, green, generally rounded or oval, and have two points projecting from the surface. The plant stems are squarish and hairy.

Uses: The AED provides a long list of maladies and ailments for which heliotrope is used. A selection from this list includes cough, eczema, fever, leprosy, rheumatism, and warts. It is also reported as a folk remedy for cancer, as a medication to induce abortions, and as a treatment for scorpion stings (AED). The latter is almost certainly a case of Doctrine of Signatures due to this plants scorpioid inflorescence. Members of certain lepidopteran families (Ithomiidae, Danaidae, and Sesiidae) are often found feeding at these flowers. Helioptrope provides pyrolizidine alkaloids which are used as defensive chemicals by some and as precursors to sex pheromones for others.

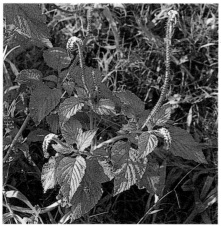

Fig. 88   The shape of heliotrope's inflorescence resembles a scorpion's tail.

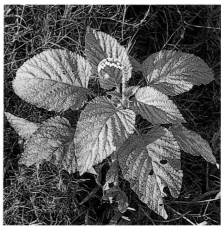

Fig. 89   Looking down on the wrinkled,
crenulate leaves of a heliotrope plant.

Blood 'Mushroom'
Aguajillo

Latin Name: *Helosis guyannensis* L.C. Rich.
Balanophoraceae: Balanophora Family

Description: The blood 'mushroom' is not a true mushroom nor member of the fungi kingdom, but actually belongs to the higher plants or angiosperms. It is a root parasite that completely lacks chlorophyll and is generally similar in habit and appearance to the plant Indian pipes (*Monotropa uniflora*) that grows in the United States. The blood 'mushroom' has a subterranean rhizome that connects to the root of its host tree. The only visible or above-ground portion of the plant is the flower stalk and inflorescence. The inflorescence is elliptical in shape, about 3-5cm long, and covered with six-sided scales. Both it, and the 5-15cm long bare stalk that bears it, are usually red in color. However, they may also be pink or brown. This plant is common in Amazonian lowlands where it often grows in clumps of several closely-spaced stalks among the leaf litter of the forest floor.

Uses: The primary indigenous use of the blood 'mushroom' is as an astringent, or to staunch the flow of blood. Both the juice of the plant and a powder made from the dried, ground material are reported as having styptic properties (SAR). It is proposed that this usage is based on a Doctrine of Signatures due to the fact that the plant is usually blood red in color (SAR). Some tribes also use it in a brew to treat diarrhea and dysentery (SAR).

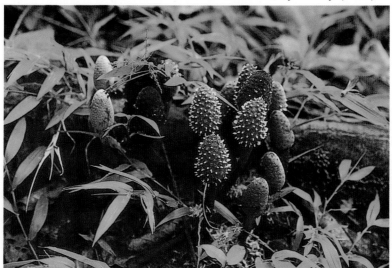

Fig. 90   A typical clump of blood 'mushrooms' (*Helosis guyannensis*).

Rubber
Shiringa

Latin Name: *Hevea brasiliensis* (Willd. ex A. Juss.) Muell.-Arg.
Euphorbiaceae: Spurge Family

Description: Rubber comes from a medium-sized tree that is native to Brazil and which grows wild in the Amazon Basin. The key characteristic for which this plant is known is the white milky latex that is produced when cut or injured. This gummy substance most likely evolved as a method to close wounds and to protect against wood-boring insects. The leaves of the rubber tree are alternately arranged and compound, with three equally-sized leaflets. Each leaflet is oval to lanceolate with an entire margin and terminates in a point. The flowers are small, white, inconspicuous, and borne in clusters. The fruits are divided into three parts which pop apart (= explosive dehiscence) when mature to disperse the seeds.

Uses: All of us are familiar with the product known as rubber (= *caucho* in Spanish) which is produced from the latex exuded by this tree. The word 'rubber' itself comes from the use of the material in the 1800's to 'rub' out mistakes written on paper with a lead pencil. Natural gum erasers are still preferred by many artists. Early use of the latex by Amazonian Indians included making waterproof pouches and bags. Some even dipped their feet in the collected latex, held them in the smoke of a fire to coagulate it, and had a waterproof shoe of sorts. Indigenous people also cooked and ate the seeds.

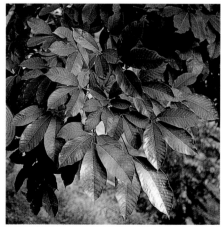

Fig. 91   Typical trifoliate leaves of a rubber tree. (Photo by Walter Judd)

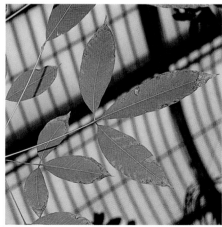

Fig. 92   The trifoliate leaves of the rubber tree. (Photo by Andrew McRobb)

Certain piranha and fruit-eating fish consume rubber seeds as part of their diet during the high-water season when the river floods and normally dry areas of forest become inundated.

Commercial development of the rubber industry started in the 1820's, but reached its peak in the Amazon Basin from 1880-1910. During these thirty years, Amazonian Indians were used as conscript labor to harvest the latex from wild trees. The Amazon rubber trade collapsed around 1915 when plantation-grown rubber trees of the same species in Southeast Asia out-produced wild-collected rubber from South America. Disease prevented rubber from being cultivated successfully in plantations in the Amazon Basin. The leading rubber producers today are Malaysia, Indonesia, and Thailand.

Rubber is harvested by making a thin, oblique cut through the bark along the trunk of the tree. The initial flow of latex lasts 3-4 hours. Trees may be tapped as frequently as every other day and have a useful life of 25 years. The dripping latex is collected in bowls, deposited in vats, and mixed with acid to coagulate it. Further processing depends on the application.

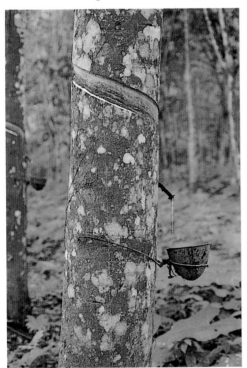

Fig. 93   A rubber tree freshly cut to induce the flow of latex.

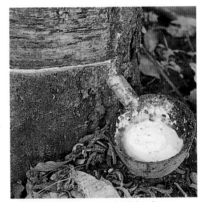

Fig. 94   Rubber latex draining into a gourd-like receptacle.

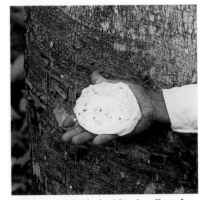

Fig. 95   A 'plug' of rubber is collected from each tree periodically.

Himatanthus
Bellaco Caspi

Latin Name: *Himatanthus sucuuba* (Spruce) Woods.
Apocynaceae: Dogbane Family

Description: This genus contains 6-7 species of medium-sized to large trees found in rainforests from Central America to northern South America. They are closely related to the genus *Plumeria* (page 103) both with respect to the appearance of the leaves and the presence of a milky white latex. The long slender leaves are simple, entire, alternate, and lanceolate in shape. They are arranged in a whorled manner which makes them resemble *Mangifera indica* (page 75) slightly, as well as *Plumeria*. The mature leaves are 25-30cm long by 3-5cm wide and come to an obvious, although somewhat blunted, point. The leaf narrows at the base to a short petiole of 2-3cm. There is an obvious yellow midvein, with very distinctive almost circular secondary veins that fork and loop back on one another. The branches have large, noticeable leaf scars present. Flowers and fruits are similar to those found in *Plumeria*.

Uses: Certain Indian tribes use the latex and/or the bark, in one form or another, to treat wounds (both fresh and persistent) (SAR). It is also used by indigenous people to suffocate and kill the larvae of the human bot fly (*Dermatobia hominis*), whose maggots develop beneath the skin of man and other mammals. Latex may also be used to treat tumors, hernias, and back pains (AED). Preparations of the latex promote the healing of broken bones (AMP). A brew of the bark provides treatments for lung ailments (BDS).

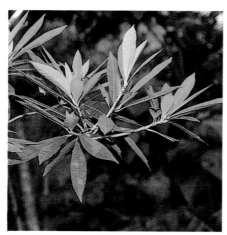

Fig. 96   A cluster of leaves of the tree
Himatanthus sucuuba.

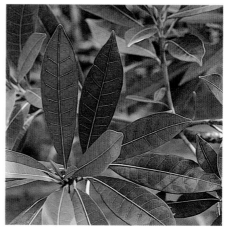

Fig. 97   Close-up of several leaves showing the
distinctive venation of *Himatanthus sucuuba.*

Ice Cream Bean
Guaba, Shimbillo

Latin Name: ***Inga edulis*** **Mart.**
Mimosaceae: Mimosa Family

Description: The genus *Inga* contains more than 350 species. Many are medium-sized trees found throughout the forests of Central and South America. The alternate leaves of *Inga* are large and distinctive, and even pinnately compound. The leaflets occur in pairs and the rachis of the leaf is noticeably widened between each pair. In *I. edulis*, mature leaves are 35-45cm long by 15-20cm wide with the petiole swollen and rounded at the base. Individual leaflets are 12-15cm long by 5-6cm wide, lanceolate and pointed, numbering 8-10 per leaf.   A large cup-like gland (extra-floral nectary) is located on the rachis between the bases of each pair of leaflets. The white inflorescences of *Inga* are globose and much like those of *Mimosa*, but vary in size and the way in which they arise from the plant. The fruit of *I. edulis* is a long (60-75cm) pod-like bean that hangs from a woody, dark brown stalk 8-10cm in length. This bean has longitudinal ridges and may be twisted.

Uses: Several dozen species of *Inga* bear edible fruit, and are cultivated for that reason, as well as for shade and ornamental value. The pod of the ice cream bean tree is packed with large dark seeds surrounded by a tasty white pulp that is eaten. Both the bark and the seeds are sometimes used by natives to treat children with dysentery (AMP). Other indigenous groups use the latex of one species to fix dyes in various materials (SAR). Several Indian tribes use the white fruit pulp for wiping the eyes and to clean the teeth (SAR).

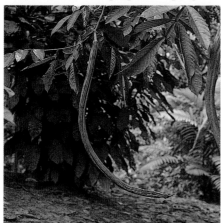

Fig. 98   The long fruit pod of the ice cream bean tree.

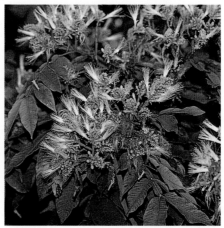

Fig. 99   The flowers and leaves of the ice cream bean tree.

Sweet Potato
Camote

Latin Name: *Ipomoea batatas* **(L.) Lam.**
Convolvulaceae: Morning Glory Family

Description: The sweet potato is native to the Andes Mountains of South America. It is a trailing perennial vine when grown in the tropics. It is often referred to as a yam, but is not a true yam which belongs to an entirely different and unrelated family (Dioscoreaceae). The leaves are simple and alternate, usually 8-10cm long by 6-8cm wide, with the new growth tightly appressed. The shape of the leaf varies from broadly triangular to somewhat star-shaped with several large pointed lobes to cordate. It produces a typical morning glory flower that is blue and white in color and about 5cm long. Stems lie on the ground, with roots produced from the nodes where the leaves emerge. Below ground is the large root or sweet potato which is elongate, asymmetrical, orange-brown in color, and about 15-20cm long.

Uses: Sweet potatoes are edible and grown throughout the world, where they are also used to make wine and alcohol, as well as food for livestock. China is currently the world's largest producer. Sweet potatoes are cultivated by indigenous groups in Malaysia, New Guinea, and Polynesia, where they form part of the staple diet. The potato may be grated and the pulpy mass applied to the skin to eliminate itching and irritations (AMP). Sweet potatoes are also used for treating asthma, burns, diarrhea, fever, nausea, and stomach problems (AED).

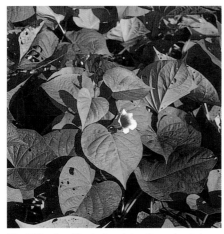

Fig. 100   A cultivated variety of sweet potato.

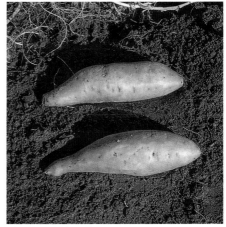

Fig. 101   The underground root or sweet potato.

Cypress Vine
Enredadera

Latin Name: *Ipomoea quamoclit* L.
Convolvulaceae: Morning Glory Family

Description: This plant is a very atypical morning glory in appearance. It is a slender, weedy herbaceous vine with very feathery, almost fern-like leaves. The leaves are alternate and very deeply divided with each individual pinna reduced to a linear, stem-like structure about half a millimeter in diameter and 2-3cm long. The entire leaf is 8-10cm long and 5-6cm wide and may have a total of 20-40 pinnae that decrease in length as they approach the tip. The showy bright red flowers are trumpet-shaped, 3-4cm long by 1-2cm in diameter, and occur singly or in small clusters. They are borne on 6-8cm long stalks from the leaf axils. When mature, the fruits are light brown, oval, papery capsules with a long slender point on the tip. They are 1-1.5cm long and about a centimeter in diameter at the base. They contain four black seeds.

Uses: This plant is often cultivated as an ornamental. Among the ailments treated with preparations from this plant are snakebite, sores, constipation, and inflammation due to the discharge of mucous membranes (DAW).

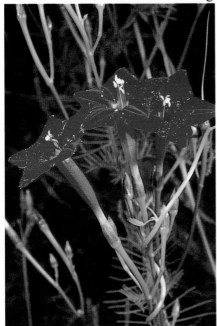

Fig. 102   The scarlet trumpet-shaped flowers of cypress vine.

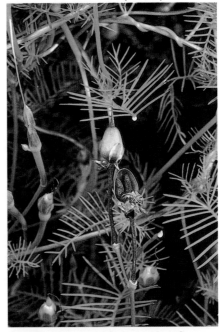

Fig. 103   The opened fruit capsule and leaves of cypress vine.

Belly Palm, Stilt Palm
Huacrapona, Barrigón

Latin Name: *Iriartea deltoidea* R. & P.
Arecaceae: Palm Family

Description: These palms grow in tropical Latin America in a variety of habitats. It is a large palm, reaching 25m high and 30cm diameter. At ground level it might be mistaken for *Socratea exorrhiza* (page 117), another common Amazonian stilt palm. However, the stilt roots of the belly palm may be as long as 180cm, but are not densely covered with spines as in the genus *Socratea*. Also, the 'root cone' formed by these closely-spaced stilt roots is dense, impossible or difficult to see through. There is usually a significant swelling about half way up the trunk of the palm. The large pinnate leaves may be 5-6m long and have irregular leaflets that are widest towards the base. The inflorescences are borne from large (1-2m), horn-shaped, hanging buds. The fruits are round, yellow-green, and 2-3cm in diameter. (HGB).

Uses: This palm is used in house construction, primarily flooring. Indians use the leaf petiole to fashion darts for their blowguns (AED). The swollen trunk area is sometimes used as a temporary canoe and as coffins (HGB).

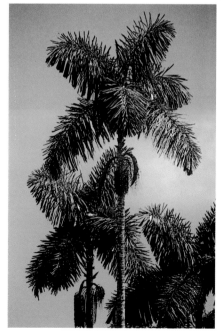

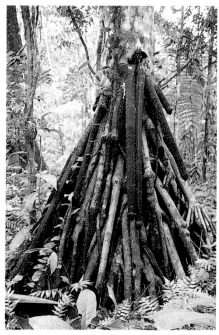

Fig. 104   The leaf crown of the belly palm.
(Photo by Paul Donahue)

Fig. 105   The dense root cone of the belly palm.   (Photo by Paul Donahue)

Physic Nut
Piñón Blanco

Latin Name: *Jatropha curcas* L.
Euphorbiaceae: Spurge Family

Description: Physic nut grows as a shrub or small tree usually less than five meters in height. The specimens examined had erect stems/trunks with leaves arranged whorl-like around all sides and from top to bottom. These characters gave the shrub a 'full' but narrow appearance. The leaves are simple and alternate, approximately as wide as they are long, with a surface that is somewhat folded and not flat. The leaves have 6-8 shallow lobes and range in size from 8-15cm long by 8-15cm wide with palmate venation. The petioles are 6-16cm long and leave a noticeable scar on the stem. The flowers are borne in clusters and are white to light green with yellow stamens. They are about one centimeter long by one centimeter in diameter. The fruits are oval to roundish, 3-4cm long, and attached to a stalk 12-15cm long.

Uses: This plant has a variety of medicinal uses but is also cultivated as an ornamental. Among the indigenous applications are to steep the leaves in water which is used to bathe people suffering from fever (SAR). The same preparation with the addition of the leaves of *Petiverea alliacea* (page 97) is used to bathe the head to relieve headache (SAR). The raw seeds have been used as a laxative (AED). Leaves are sometimes applied in poultice form to treat infection (AED). The latex is used to relieve toothache pain (GMJ) and to treat sore gums in children (SAR). A decoction of the leaves is used similarly to barbasco to kill fish, while the seeds are a source of oil (AED).

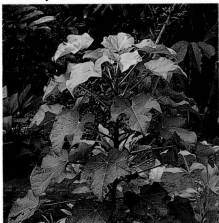

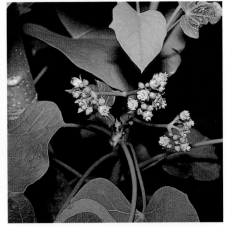

Fig. 106   The stem and leaves of a young physic nut plant.

Fig. 107   Blossoms of the physic nut plant.

Black Physic Nut
Piñón Negro

Latin Name: *Jatropha gossypifolia* L.
Euphorbiaceae: Spurge Family

Description: Black physic nut grows as a woody shrub, seldom getting more than 2-3 meters in height. The foliage is very distinctive with the shiny new growth having a deep red to almost black color, while the older leaves are a dark smoky green. Most leaves have three finger-like lobes (some have five) and are approximately 10-12cm long by 10-12cm wide. The leaves are simple, alternate and borne on 10-12cm long petioles. The venation is palmate and the leaf margins are finely dentate. Flowers have five red petals and a yellow center. They are borne in small clusters at the end of stalks at the tip of the central stem. The open, bell-shaped (= campanulate) blossoms are approximately 1cm long by 1.5-2cm in diameter. The bright green fruits are squarish, barrel-shaped and about 3-4cm long by 2-3cm in diameter. The surface is smooth, but the entire fruit is grooved into longitudinal sections. Dark red triangular leafy structures at the base of the flowers persist at the base of the fruits. The edges are lined with many, tiny, regularly-spaced yellow knobs, as are the margins of the leaves and the new growth branches.

Uses: This shrub is often cultivated for its showy foliage, flowers, and fruit. The latex is used to treat burns and hemorrhoids (AED), as well as to promote the healing of wounds (BDS). Various Indian groups use extracts as purgatives and to induce vomiting (AED). Macerated leaves are applied in poultice form for headaches (RAR) and for swellings (SOU).

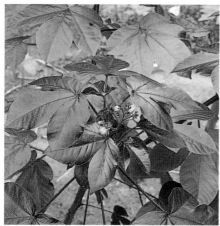

Fig. 108   Leaves, fruits, and flowers of the black physic nut.

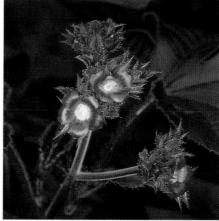

Fig. 109   Close-up of the flowers of the black physic nut.

Air Plant
Hoja de Aire

Latin Name: *Kalanchoe pinnata* (Lam.) Pers.
Crassulaceae: Stonecrop Family

Description: The genus *Kalanchoe* is primarily African and Asian in distribution, normally inhabiting dry habitats. Air plant is an introduced species which has become naturalized in tropical lowland forest habitats. This herbaceous plant has thick, succulent leaves that are opposite and pinnate. The margins of the leaves are edged with dark red or purple and have regular shallow indentations giving it a scalloped appearance. There are typically three leaflets per leaf, the two lateral ones of equal size and the central one considerably larger. Mature leaflets are 6-8cm long by 4-5cm wide. The entire leaf is borne on long fleshy purple petiole 8-12cm long. Fallen leaves take root from the scalloped edges resulting in the common name 'life everlasting' that is used for air plant in Belize (AAB). The inflorescence is a panicle that consists of a large numbers of pendent flowers on a tall stalk that is higher than the plant itself (seldom more than a meter). The green and purple flowers are tubular, about 2-3cm in length by 5-8mm in diameter.

Uses: The air plant is both cultivated as an ornamental and used for treating a wide range of illnesses. Taken in ways that vary from an application of heated leaves to drinking a tea, SAR recount its use for treating boils, internal bruises and broken bones, and intestinal problems. It is also used for headache, earache, fever, heartburn and various inflammations (AED), as well as for eye irritations, bronchitis, and to promote the healing of sores (RVM).

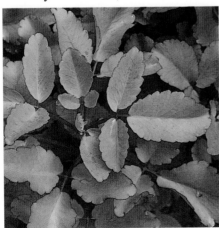

Fig. 110   Leaves of the air plant.

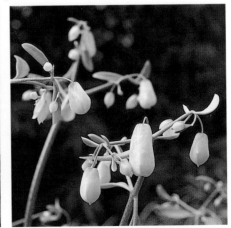

Fig. 111   Inflorescences of the air plant.

Lantana
Aya Albaca

Latin Name: *Lantana camara* L.
Verbenaceae: Vervain or Teak Family

Description: Lantana is a weedy herb usually found in disturbed areas that can become climbing or sometimes develop into a woody shrub. It is typically 1-2m high, and has squarish stems that are often covered with prickles. The leaves are simple and opposite, emerging from each node at right angles to the leaves of the node nearest it. The leaf edge is regularly serrate, while the surface is wrinkled and has a rough texture (= scabrous). When the leaves or stems are crushed, a distinctive pungent, recognizable odor is given off. The leaf shape is broadly lanceolate to cordate with a pointed tip, while they range in size from 8-10cm long by 3-5cm wide, with a 2-3cm petiole. The color of the inflorescence varies greatly with mixtures of red, pink, orange, and yellow. Inflorescences consist of dense round heads (3-5cm in diameter) composed of 10-25 flowers. Each blossom has a long tubular base and widely flaring petals at the apex. The heads are on 5-10cm long stalks. The smooth, round fruits occur in ball-like clusters 2-3cm in diameter. They begin green but turn blue-black to black with maturity.

Uses: The leaves of lantana are used to relieve itching (AAB) and are mixed with other plants for respiratory problems including cough and bronchitis (AED). A leaf decoction is used to treat rheumatism and stomach problems (SOU) as well as colds and fever (AED). The plant is mixed in water to bathe anemic children (RVM) and for use as a sedative bath (AED).

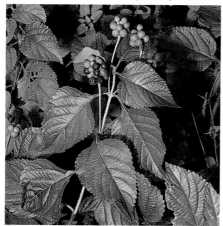

Fig. 112   Leaves and fruit of lantana.

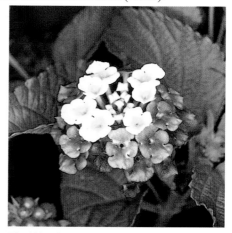

Fig. 113   Close-up of flower of lantana.

Santa Maria
Santa María

Latin Name: *Lepianthes peltata* **(L.) Raf.**
Piperaceae: Pepper Family

Description: This species with the common name Santa Maria, may also
be found listed as *Piper peltatum* (AED) or *Pothomorphe peltata* (AHG,
TBC). It is a shrubby succulent herb up to two meters in height that is
commonly found in disturbed areas. It has large, alternate, simple, entire
leaves that are nearly round or heart-shaped (= cordate) with a short point at
the tip. The upper surface of the leaf is darker and appears wrinkled, while
the under surface is light green to almost white. The petiole is 10-20cm long
and does not attach to the leaf at the base, but rather about a third of the way
in from the margin (= peltate, hence the species name). The palmate veins
radiating out from the attachment point are easily visible. The leaves typically
range from 15-25cm in diameter. The petiole is laterally-flattened and thick at
its base. The flower stalk emerges from the top of the petiole (which is
grooved) near the stem (= axillary). It bears a cluster of 3-8 light green spikes
7-10cm long with tiny reduced flowers characteristic of this family.

Uses: A leaf decoction of Santa Maria has been used to increase urine flow,
relieve fever, and induce vomiting (AED), and is reported to induce abortions
(SAR). Different preparations are also used to reduce inflammation, eliminate
intestinal worms, and treat burns, colds, swellings, headaches, and toothaches
(JAD, RVM, DAW). It has been used by some groups to both kill fish and
lice (JAD) and to keep away ticks (DAW). Food is wrapped in the leaves.

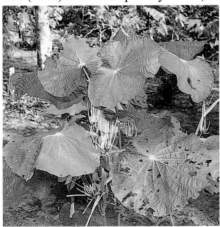

Fig. 114   The peltate leaf of Santa Maria.

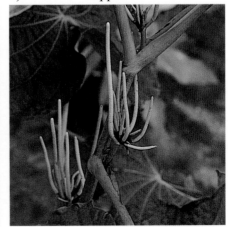

Fig. 115   A cluster of flower/fruit stalks of
Santa Maria.

Thatch Palm
Irapay

Latin Name: *Lepidocaryum tenue* Mart.
Arecaceae: Palm Family

Description: This palm is listed as *Lepidocaryum tessmannii*, a synonym, in the AED. It is a small, slender, understory palm found throughout tropical South America, especially in western Amazonia. It is typically 2-4 meters tall with a ringed trunk and seldom gets greater than 3-4cm in diameter. There are usually twenty leaves or less that are borne on long slender petioles. The leaves are palmate and deeply split into halves, then further subdivided into long, narrow leaflets that range from 50-75cm long by 2-8cm wide (HGB). The total number of leaflets per leaf can vary from 4-22 (HGB). The barrel-shaped fruits are 2-3cm long by 1-2cm in diameter and covered with tightly overlapping orange-brown scales. These palms reproduce vegetatively from underground stems (= rhizomes) which sometimes results in many being found clustered in one area.

Uses: As the English common name implies, this palm is used in the construction of roof thatch. The palm leaves are cut, including the petiole, then woven together and tied to a slat about two meters in length. The fin-ished thatch section (= *crisneja*) is then dried in the sun. Successive layers of *crisnejas* are attached in an overlapping manner to support poles by means of philodendron roots. The life expectancy of this kind of roofing material is about five years. Roofs constructed of thatch palm cover the majority of *Ribereños* dwellings along the Amazon and Napo Rivers.

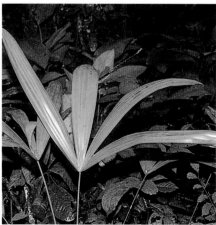

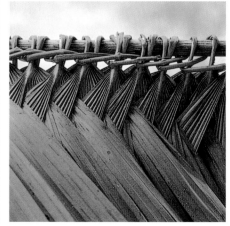

Fig. 116 ⋅ The deeply split leaf of thatch palm, a small understory palm.

Fig. 117   A section of newly-woven roof thatch or *crisneja* using thatch palm leaves.

Lippia
Pampa Orégano

Latin Name: *Lippia alba* (Mill.) N.E.Br.
Verbenaceae: Vervain or Teak Family

Description: This species is 1-2m in height with a very straggly, weedy overall appearance. There are many slender, sparsely foliated woody stems. The leaves are extremely similar to those of *Lantana camara* (page 70), although there seems to be considerably more space between the nodes. The leaves are simple and opposite, with the margins distinctly serrate. The surface of the leaves has a wrinkled appearance. They are ovate to lanceolate, narrowing towards the tip. Average size is about 5-8cm long by 2-3 cm wide, with a short petiole. At some nodes tiny miniature pairs of leaves are present. The small pink axillary flowers are very similar in form to those of *L. camara*, but occur in smaller clusters. The leaves when crushed have a strong but pleasing aroma to them.

Uses: A preparation of the leaves of *Lippia alba* placed in water is given to women about to give birth in order to accelerate the delivery of the baby (AMP). This mixture is also supposed to eliminate the pain of childbirth (AMP). Traditional healers or *curanderos* use this and other plants combined as a bath during ceremonies (AED). The crushed leaves in water are also used to bathe the head as a treatment for headaches (SAR). More than one indigenous group uses this plant for stomachaches (RVM, BDS). A leaf decoction is also used as a calmant and as a sedative (GMJ).

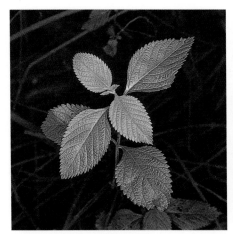

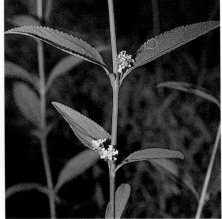

Fig. 118   Leaves of *Lippia alba*.   Fig. 119   Leaves and flowers of *Lippia alba*.

Toothache Tree
Insira Amarilla

Latin Name: *Maclura tinctoria* (L.) Gaud.
Moraceae: Fig or Mulberry Family

Description: The toothache tree is a large monoecious canopy tree that has spiny branches and a milky latex. The alternate, simple leaves have toothed margins and obvious drip-tips. The venation is distinctive. The trunk has raised reddish pustules (AHG). The female (= pistillate) flowers occur in compact rounded inflorescences on very short stalks from the branches. The male (= staminate) flowers are arranged along elongated spikes (= catkins). The fruits are multiples of drupelets with accessory tissue.

Uses: As the English common name implies, this tree is often used to treat problems associated with toothaches. Indigenous people collect the latex on 'cotton' provided by the balsa tree *Ochroma pyrimidale* (page 88) or by kapok trees *Ceiba* spp. (page 34), and then apply it to the infected tooth (AED). In this manner, the removal of the tooth is accomplished without pain and bleeding, but care must be exercised as this technique will evidently remove healthy teeth with equal ease (NIC). Preparations of this tree are also used as a diuretic and to treat venereal problems (AED). The AED also suggests that due to certain chemicals produced by this tree that it would serve as an astringent and antiseptic. It is further used for cough, gout, sore throat, and rheumatism (RAR). It is the source of an olive-colored dye, and the wood is used for lumber and in carpentry (AED).

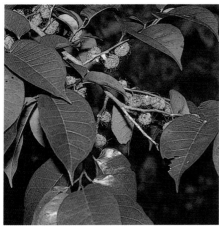

Fig. 120 Leaves and fruits of the toothache tree (*Maclura tinctoria*).

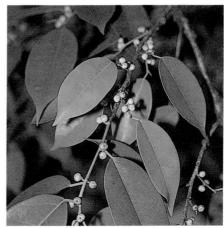

Fig. 121 Leaves and fruits of the toothache tree (*Maclura tinctoria*).

Mango
Mango

Latin Name: *Mangifera indica* L.
Anacardiaceae: Sumac or Poison Ivy Family

Description: Mango is a large dark evergreen tree native to India, but now naturalized and cultivated throughout the tropical areas of the world. It may reach a height of 40 meters, but is often much smaller. Wild mango trees inhabit secondary lowland forest habitats. The simple, entire, alternate leaves are long and narrow and come to a point. They are typically 20-30cm long by 2-6cm wide. The petioles range from very short to a length of five centimeters. There is a distinct yellow midvein and obvious secondary veins nearly perpendicular to it. The leaves are arranged in whorl-like clusters at the ends of the branches giving them an almost star-like appearance. The inflorescence is a branched pyramidal panicle occuring at the ends of branches and containing large clusters of small flowers. Mango fruits vary greatly in size (5-30cm), shape, and color according to the variety. Fruit colors include red, green, purple, yellow, and pink. Some fruits are almost round, while others are oval and asymmetrical. They are borne in small groups from hanging stalks 20-50cm long.

Uses: Mango is cultivated as a shade tree and for its edible fruit which is eaten raw, canned, or used in the making of pickles and chutneys. It is a popular tropical tree because it does well on poor soils. Some Indian groups use varying dosages of a brew of the leaves as a contraceptive and to induce abortion (SAR). Flowers are used as an antiasthmatic or expectorant (VDF).

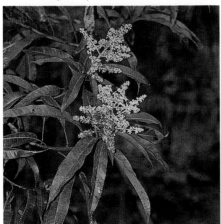

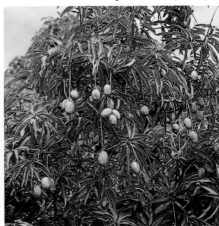

Fig. 1   A star-like cluster of mango leaves with flowers at the end of the branch.

Fig. 2   Clusters of mango fruits hanging from fruit stalks.

Cassava, Manioc
Yuca

Latin Name: *Manihot esculenta* Crantz.
Euphorbiaceae: Spurge Family

Description: Cassava is an erect shrub with a straight slender stalk that can sometimes reach three meters in height. It is much more commonly seen growing at heights of 1-2 meters. As the plant matures, the lower part of the stem becomes knobby. The leaves are simple, alternate, and palmate with typically 3-5 deep finger-like lobes. The underside of the leaf appears white due to a waxy covering. The leaves are 15-25cm long and equally wide. They are borne on long (15-30cm), often red petioles. The small yellow-green flowers are borne in clusters and are seldom bigger than 1-2cm. The roots are large brown starchy tubers that sometimes reach 60cm in length. They look like dark sweet potatoes (page 64). Removal of the fibrous brown exterior reveals a hard white interior like a potato. This plant contains a milky latex.

Uses: Cassava is indigenous to Tropical America, but is now grown all over the tropics. It is one of the staple crops for subsistence farmers and the primary source of carbohydrate in South America. The roots contain cyanide which is removed when they are cooked or heated. The starchy tubers are often ground into a flour that is used to make 'cakes' and tapioca pudding. The roots may also be boiled, baked, roasted, or toasted. Cassava tubers are used in making alcoholic beverages such as *masato*, which involves chewing the root and spitting it into a large pot where the saliva initiates the fermentation.

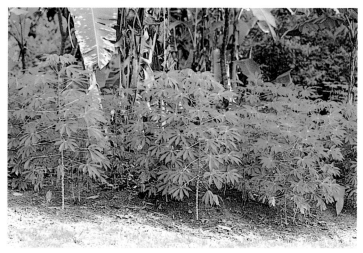

Fig. 124   A stand of cassava planted along the Amazon River, Peru.

Medicinally and culturally, cassava has a variety of uses besides food. Juice from the grated tubers for example has been used directly to wash the head as a treatment for scabies, mixed with water and taken for diarrhea, and when extracted from the cultivated strain with highest cyanide content (*yuca brava*), directly as a fish poison (SAR). One Indian group uses the leaves in the form of a poultice to staunch the flow of blood (AED). Others use the starch with rum and apply it topically to children with skin problems (AED). Additionally, various preparations of cassava have been used in the treatment of fever and chills (RVM), sterile women (AED), and for sore muscles (GMJ).

Many varieties or cultivars of cassava exist, some of which are extremely poisonous. Indigenous peoples have invented ingenious methods for dealing with this. Some cultivars high in cyanide are 'processed' by grating the tuber on a flat board with resin-embedded rocks on it. The wet pulp is then put in a long, banana-shaped woven basket which is hung by a loop from a support. The basket is pulled or twisted resulting in the cyanide-containing liquid exiting the holes of the weave and leaving the edible material behind.

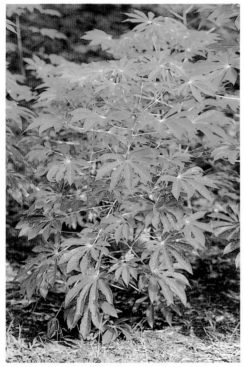

Fig. 125   The palmate leaves and long petioles give cassava plants a very distinctive appearance.

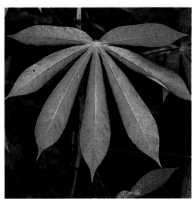

Fig. 126   Close up of the distinctive palmate leaf of the cassava plant.

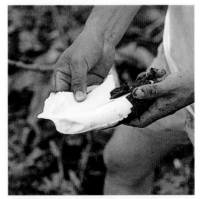

Fig. 127   The large starchy underground tuber of the cassava plant.

Chewing Gum Tree
Sapodilla

Latin Name: *Manilkara zapota* (L.) Van Royen
Sapotaceae: Sapodilla Family

Description: This is a tree of medium size (15-20m) native to Central America, but now cultivated in tropical regions throughout the world. The simple, alternate leaves are arranged in spiral clusters at the ends of the branches. Leaves are slender and generally ovate terminating in a blunt point. They range from 6-12cm long by 2-5cm wide, with a 2-4cm long petiole. The midvein is distinctive and appears recessed while the secondary venation is barely discernible. The light-colored flowers are approximately 1cm long by .5cm in diameter and are borne on stalks of the same length or slightly greater. Both bud and stalk are covered with light brown hair and occur in small groups at the branch apices among the leaf petioles. The flowers do not open widely. The large round berries produced are light brown in color, approximately 6-8cm in diameter, and have a rough surface. They are borne on short (1-2cm) stout stalks that are woody and almost appear to be a continuation of the branch.

Uses: This tree is widely cultivated for its edible fruits which are produced year round. Its white milky sap is called *chicle*, which was the source of commercial chewing gum and the origin of the product 'chiclet'. This latex was obtained by tapping the tree in a manner similar to tapping rubber by men called *chicleros*. It was chewed by Mayan Indians before the arrival of the Spaniards, and was once investigated as a potential rubber substitute.

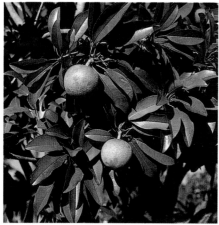

Fig. 128   Fruit and leaves of the chewing gum tree (*Manilkara zapota*).

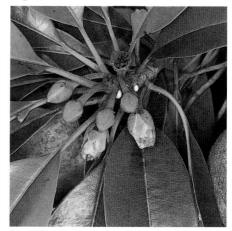

Fig. 129   Close-up of the flowers of the chewing gum tree (*Manilkara zapota*).

Wild Garlic
Ajo Sacha

Latin Name: *Mansoa alliacea* (Lam.) A.Gentry
Bignoniaceae: Trumpet Vine or Catalpa Family

Description: This plant is a climbing vine or forest liana that has a distinctive garlic-like odor when crushed or cut. Wild garlic has compound, opposite leaves that are composed of two equal-sized symmetrical leaflets. Each leaflet is oval and entire, terminating in an obvious drip-tip. In the cultivated specimen examined, the leaflets were approximately 7-8cm long by 2-3cm wide. However, older naturally-growing specimens are reported at 2-3 times that size. There are glands present at the base of the leaflets. The leaflets are borne on petioles and have a distinctive looping secondary venation where the veins do not reach the margin but rather turn back towards the midvein and connect with adjacent secondary veins. Some tendrils are present, both simple and with a 3-part tip (= trifid), which arise from between the leaflets. The lavender flowers are large and trumpet-shaped, borne in clusters. The fruit is a capsule that is bean-like in shape.

Uses: Wild garlic bark is mixed with water and used as a bath for people with asthma or who smoke excessively (AMP). Bark raspings taken orally with water, or with sugarcane rum are used to treat asthma and arthritis, respectively (AMP). The most common form of usage seems to be parts of the plant in water which is used to bathe oneself and treat or protect against: evil spirits (AED), fever (GMJ), influenza and aches and pains (BDS), as well as nervousness, fatigue, and cramps (AED).

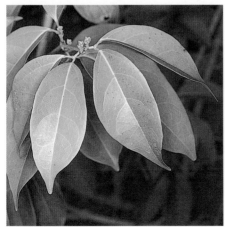

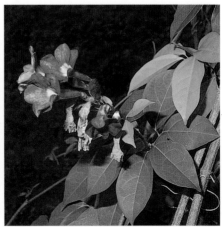

Fig. 130   The opposite compound leaves of wild garlic.

Fig. 131   Flowers of wild garlic.

Capinuri
Capinurí

Latin Name: *Maquira coriacea* (Karst.) C. Berg.
Moraceae: Fig or Mulberry Family

Description: The capinuri is an emergent tree found in swampy habitats throughout the Amazon Basin. Large buttresses that may reach 5-6m in height are present at the base of the trunk. The bark exudes a cream-colored latex when cut or injured. The simple, alternate leaves are oval and pointed, but seldom seen at ground level. Their edges are entire and unbroken. Small globose flowers form in the leaf axil. One of the most distinctive features of this tree is the realistic phallic shape exhibited by the ends of its fallen branches. This is caused when the penis-like tip of the branch breaks away from the cup-like receptacle it has grown from. These branches have resulted in a vulgar, rhyming nickname.

Uses: Capinuri latex is used to treat dislocations, hernias, and backaches (AED). Local vendors state that capinuri can be used to increase virility, a classic example of Doctrine of Signatures. The lumber is used in the production of plywood (AED). A narcotic snuff is made from a related tree (SAR).

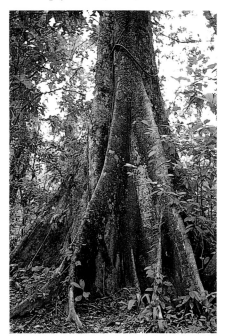
Fig. 132   The buttressed trunk of a capinuri tree.

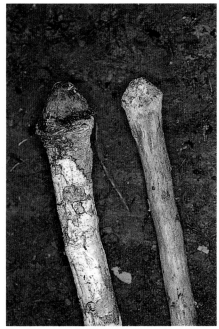
Fig. 133   The phallic-shaped branches of the capinuri tree.

Moriche Palm
Aguaje

Latin Name: *Mauritia flexuosa* L.
Arecaceae: Palm Family

Description: The moriche palm is commonly found in swampy habitats within the New World tropics, and is often seen growing along riverbanks. Moriche is a large (12-15m), generally solitary palm with a stout (30-50cm diameter) trunk. The leaves are fan-like, with a petiole that continues through the blade as a midrib (= costapalmate). The leaves are 2-2.5m long by 4-4.5m wide and may be up to 20 in number (HGB). The blade of the leaf is deeply cleft in half, with the halves further divided into long narrow leaflets that have small spines along their edges. There may be as many as 200 leaflets per leaf, the tips of which tend to spread out in a plane different from the rest of the leaf. The inflorescences are large (>2 meters) and composed of many small flowers on hanging parallel branches. The fruits are cylindrical or barrel-shaped, about 5-8cm long and 4-5cm in diameter. They are covered with reddish brown to purple scales which are about .5cm in diameter. When the scales are removed, a bright yellow-orange inner pulp is revealed. Fruits are produced in great quantities on each tree, but have only one seed each.

Uses: The fruits or *aguajes* are consumed raw, as a fruit drink, or may be used to make wine or as a flavoring in ice cream. The leaves and petioles are used to fashion roof thatch, floor mats, rafts, and for their fibers (AED). In Brazil, oil is extracted from the fruits for domestic use (HGB). Fibers from the young leaves are used to make rope, hammocks, and baskets (HGB).

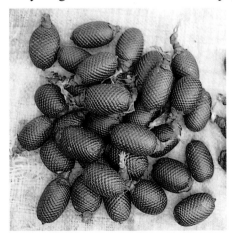

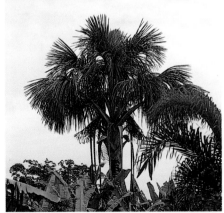

Fig. 134   Moriche palm fruits or *aguajes*.   Fig. 135   Growth habit of the moriche palm.

82

China Berry
Paraíso

Latin Name: *Melia azedarach* L.
Meliaceae: Mahogany Family

Description: China berry grows as a shrub to small tree and is native to
Asia, although it is widely cultivated outside its natural range. It has large,
odd, bipinnately compound leaves. The leaflets are usually composed of 7 or
9 pinnules. Each pinnule is lanceolate with a long pointed apex and a distinctly serrated margin. The showy flowers occur in large clusters on
branched stalks. The lavender buds open to reveal five slender white petals,
with a slender tubular-cylindrical center structure from which the yellow
anthers can be seen at its tip. The flowers are less than two centimeters in
diameter and develop into poisonous fleshy fruits (= drupes) with a pit.

Uses: The leaves of China berry are used as an insecticide, to induce
vomiting, and to reduce fevers (PEA). The bark and roots have also been
used to induce vomiting, as well as a substitute for quinine (AED). The bark
is used as an abortive and to clean external ulcers (AED). This plant has been
used to treat colds and flu, and in bath form for vitality and strength (AED).

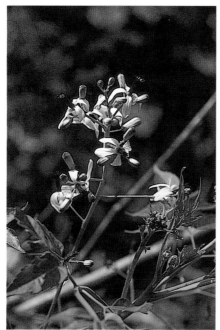

Fig. 136   The showy flowers of China berry.

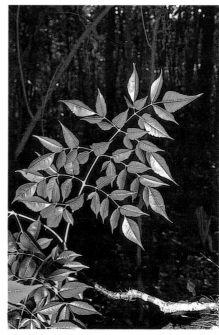

Fig. 137   The bipinnately compound leaf of
the China berry tree.

Sensitive Plant
Chami

Latin Name: *Mimosa pudica* L.
Mimosaceae: Mimosa Family

Description: The sensitive plant is a low-growing herb that seldom reaches a meter in height and often is found in disturbed areas. The leaves are even bipinnately compound with typically four finger-sized leaflets. There is a petiole 6-10cm long to which the leaflets attach without stalks. These leaflets range from 6-10cm long by 2-2.5cm wide. They are composed of many (30-50) tiny oblong pinnae that are .5-1cm long by only 1-2mm wide, giving the leaflet a feathery or fern-like appearance. The unique feature for which the plant is named is the ability of the leaflets to quickly fold up and close along their central axis, the opposing pinnae becoming appressed, in response to disturbance. The entire leaf itself will drop down towards the stem when the petiole is touched. The blossoms are pink and round, about 2cm in diameter. They are borne singly from stalks along the length of the stem, which is often armed with small thorns.

Uses: A tea from the leaves of this plant is drunk by women during menstruation as a contraceptive (AMP). A Doctrine of Signatures usage has been proposed noting that sometimes the leaves are placed in pillows to help people sleep (SAR). The leaves may also be powdered and used as a sleeping potion (AED). In Central America, sensitive plant has been used as a pain reliever, relaxant, diuretic, and antispasmodic (AAB). The dried leaves are also sometimes smoked to alleviate muscle spasms and backache (AAB).

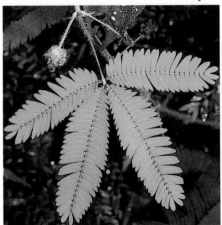

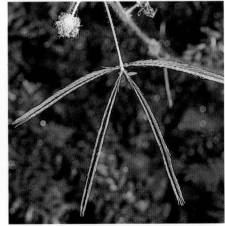

Fig. 138 The palmate-looking leaf of the sensitive plant before it is touched.

Fig. 139 The same leaf closed in response to the leaflets being touched.

Mucuna
Vaca Ñahui

Latin Name: *Mucuna rostrata* Benth.
Fabaceae: Bean or Pea Family

Description: Mucuna is a rainforest liana with alternate, compound leaves, each of which is composed of three leaflets (= trifoliate). The leaflets are asymmetrical, ovate to rhomboid in shape, have entire margins and come to an extended point. They range from 10-14cm long by 6-9cm wide (TBC). The leaves are borne on long petioles (6-10cm) that are somewhat expanded at their base (= pulvinate). The inflorescence is composed of small clusters of orange-yellow flowers that hang down from a stalk of 10-20cm length. The unusual shape of the flower is reminiscent of an open parrot's beak (JLC's interpretation), with a distinct top and bottom section. These structures also look like partial sections of dugout canoes. The longer bottom part is 6-8cm long. The hairy fruit is a curved legume 6-8cm long by 2-3cm wide.

Uses: The seeds of mucuna are prepared for use as a diuretic and as an antihemorrhoidal agent, and are also carried in case of snake bite (AED). The fruit hairs have been used as a mechanical vermifuge (SOU). The hairs that cover the legume or fruit are of an urticating or stinging nature and should not be touched.

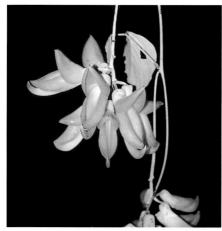

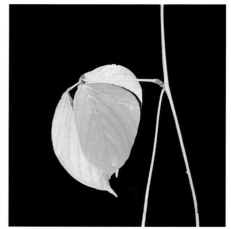

Fig. 140   The showy orange flowers of *Mucuna rostrata*.

Fig. 141   The compound trifoliate leaf of *Mucuna rostrata*.

Banana, Plantain
Banano, Plátano

Latin Name: *Musa acuminata* (cultivar) = banana
Musa acuminata X *balbisiana* (cultivar) = plantain
Musaceae: Banana Family

Description: These are herbaceous plants that become tree-like, with large alternate leaves that are simple and entire. The long (1-3m) leaves occur in a whorl at the top of the plant, and may tear into parallel strips that are attached at the midvein. The petiole and sheath of the leaf clasps the stem or trunk which may get 20-30cm in diameter. The inflorescence is a large, hanging stalk with clusters of whitish, pinkish, or reddish flowers. The fruit (the banana or plantain) is actually an elongated berry with a thick, leathery cover. Each stalk usually contains rings of fruits. There are hundreds of cultivars of the genus *Musa*. Some taxonomists previously separated bananas and plantains into two separate species: *M. sapientum* (banana) and *M. paradisiaca* (plantain). The ripened fruits of bananas are sweet and soft, while plantains are not. Mature bananas may be yellow or red in color and vary in size from 8-25cm.

Uses: Bananas and plantains are cultivated and eaten throughout the tropics, although native to Asia. Bananas are eaten fresh or lightly fried. Plantains are fried or boiled and eaten. Preparations of *Musa* are used to treat tuberculosis and pulmonary scars (AED), as well as bronchitis, cough, diarrhea, and fever (RAR). Heated banana leaves have been used to treat leishmaniasis (JAD). Plantain has been used for gout and earache (RVM).

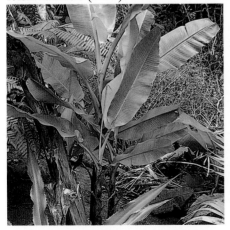

Fig. 142 Young banana plants that have been produced vegitatively from the adjacent trunk.

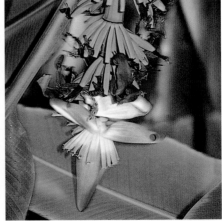

Fig. 143 A fruit stalk with banana flowers and developing fruits.

Jaboticaba
Jaboticaba

Latin Name: *Myrciaria cauliflora* (Mart.) O. Berg
Myrtaceae: Myrtle Family

Description: Under cultivated conditions, jaboticaba grows as a large shrub about 2-3m in height. It has small, simple, entire, opposite leaves that range in size from 1.5-3.5cm long to .5-1.5cm wide . They are rounded to lanceolate in shape, have a very short (2-3mm) petiole, and terminate in a point. There is a distinctive marginal vein that runs parallel to the edge, plus diagonal secondary veins with reticulate venation between them. Foliage is dense with many small opposite branches, each bearing 10-12 leaves. The flowers are small (less than a centimeter) and white, occurring in dense clusters all along the branches and trunks. The smooth round fruits are green when young but mature to shiny purple-black. They range from approximately 2-4cm in diameter and are similar to large grapes with a thin skin that surrounds a sweet white pulp. They also occur in clusters on the trunks.

Uses: This tree is widely cultivated in the tropics for its fruit which can be eaten raw, used in preserves, or made into a wine.

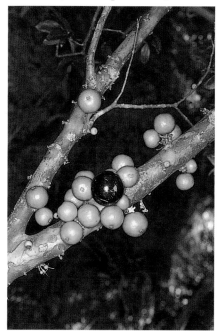

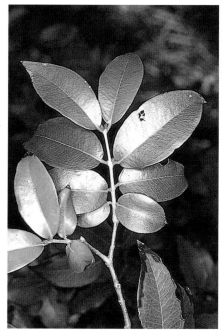

Fig. 144   The fruit and small flowers of
jaboticaba (*Myrciaria cauliflora*).

Fig. 145   The small opposite leaves of the
jaboticaba bush (*Myrciaria cauliflora*).

Camu Camu
Camu Camu

Latin Name: *Myrciaria dubia* (HBK) McVaugh
Myrtaceae: Myrtle Family

Description: Camu camu is a fruit-producing lowland tree that is indigenous to the Amazon Basin and found in abundance along the Xingu and Napo River drainages. This species is often found growing at the edges of oxbow lakes. It grows as a large bush or small tree ranging from 2-8m in height, with a slender trunk that may attain a diameter of 15cm. The leaves are simple, elongate, entire, opposite, and have distinctly pointed tips. The midvein is usually clearly visible with the secondary venation closely parallel, but difficult to see. They range in size from 4-10cm long by 2-4cm wide, and have a short petiole less than a centimeter long. Up to a dozen small white flowers are borne in the leaf axils. The round fruits are about 2-3cm in diameter and have a smooth, shiny surface that is red-purple to red and remindful of a large grape. (CFNA)

Uses: Camu camu fruits are sold for raw consumption. Like other tropical fruits, they can also be squeezed to make drinks or used to flavor other food items. In Iquitos (Peru) for example, camu camu is made into a popular ice cream. Camu camu's major benefit is its Vitamin C content, which is more than any plant (30 times as much as is in citrus). This is one of the little-known forest products that has great potential for future use, especially in the health food industry. The fruits are also an important source of food for fish of inundated forest areas.

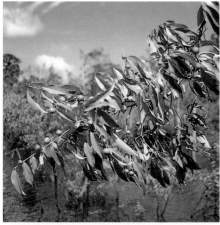
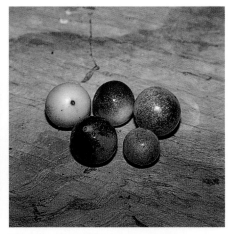

Fig. 146   Leaves and fruit of the camu camu tree. (Photo by Ghillean Prance)

Fig. 147   Fruit of the camu camu tree.

Balsa
Balsa

Latin Name: *Ochroma pyramidale* (Cav. ex Lam.) Urban
Bombacaceae: Balsa Family

Description: Balsa is a medium-sized tree ranging from 10-30 meters in height. It is common in second growth forests in areas containing richer soils. The large distinctive leaves are simple and alternately arranged, clustered at the ends of the branches. The leaves are sometimes entire and cordate, but normally have from 3-5 broad lobes. They are approximately as wide as they are long and range from 10-40cm in length. Petiole length varies greatly and may be anywhere from 5-40cm in length. Both the petioles and the underside of the leaves are covered with dense brown hair. The large white leathery flowers are formed by separate petals rolled together to form a tube. They are up to 15cm long and 5cm wide, opening at night. The long (up to 25cm) narrow fruits are smooth and black on the outside, containing many small seeds embedded in a cottony material on the inside (TBC).

Uses: The utility of balsa comes from its extremely lightweight wood. It has long been used to fashion rafts, with the word *balsa* meaning raft in Spanish. In the Amazon region, it is used for making floats for fishing nets and buoys. The tree bark has been used for cordage (AED). The cotton surrounding the aerially-dispersed seeds has been used to stuff toys (RVM). In times of high water, balsa has been used to construct floating walkways between buildings. In industrialized nations, it has been used for decades for models and crafts.

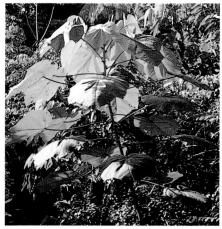

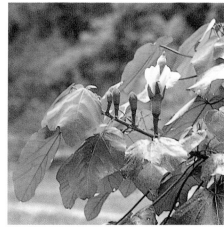

Fig. 148   The broadly lobed leaves of a young balsa tree.

Fig. 149   Leaves, buds, and flower of a balsa tree.   (Photo by Paul Donahue)

Wild Basil
Pichana Albaca

Latin Name: ***Ocimum micranthum*** **Willd.**
Lamiaceae: Mint Family

Description: Wild basil is a small, aromatic weedy herb that grows to a height of about a meter, but is often seen shorter. It has squarish stems with simple, pointed, oval-lanceolate leaves. Each leaf usually has from 16-24 teeth, irregularly spaced giving the margin an irregularly serrate appearance. Mature leaves are 5-6cm long by 2-3cm wide, with a 2-3cm long petiole. The small lavender to pink flowers are borne on upright square stalks 6-12cm long. The flowers themselves are only several millimeters long and wide, lavender on the outside with darker purple markings on the inside. They protrude from a uniquely-shaped, green, boxlike stucture (= calyx) that has a spatulate top and a bottom portion with three forward-projecting spikes. This calyx is approximately .5cm wide by 1cm long, and turns brown after the flower falls off. The flower stalk is more compacted when young, before the blossoms appear and has a distinctly pyramidal appearance at that time.

Uses: The leaves and stems of this plant give off a highly aromatic and pleasing odor when crushed, leading to its use as both a spice and a perfume (SAR). Like other aromatic plants, it is also often used in therapeutic baths, such as for the treatment of headache and fever (VDF). The liquid extracted from the crushed leaves has been used for inflammation of the eyes (SAR). A tea is also made from wild basil and used to treat the flu (AED). This plant is reported to have hallucinogenic properties (RVM).

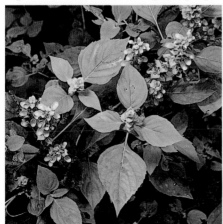

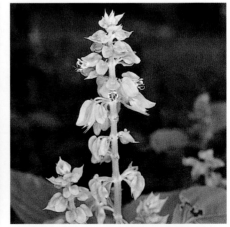

Fig. 150   Leaves and flower stalks of wild basil.

Fig. 151   Close-up of the flower stalk of wild basil showing blossom and unique calyx.

Rice
Arroz

Latin Name: *Oryza sativa* L.
Poaceae: Grass Family

Description: Rice is an aquatic plant that has evolved a specialized stem and root system which permits it to grow in standing water. Rice that is cultivated this way is called 'paddy' rice. Although rice requires large amounts of water to grow well, it does not have to be grown in standing water. Varieties that are not grown in standing water are called 'upland' rice.

Rice is a member of the grass family, as are all cereal grains such as corn, wheat, barley, and millet. Due to its long period of cultivation, it has developed into thousands of different locally-grown varieties. The following are therefore only general characteristics applicable to the plant. Rice grows in clusters of long, slender strap-like leaves that are typically 60-90cm tall. However, varieties occur that may reach heights of 3-4 meters. The plant produces many tiny white dangling flowers at the end of a stalk. This stalk will bear the rice grains which are green while developing, turning yellow or golden brown at maturity. The grains are usually 1-2cm long and number 20-60 per stalk. Cultivated rice is a common sight throughout Amazonia, where it is planted along the riverbanks as the water recedes, In appearance, it is light green and weedy-looking from a distance. When mature grains and seedheads are present, entire riverbanks and fields may have a yellow hue.

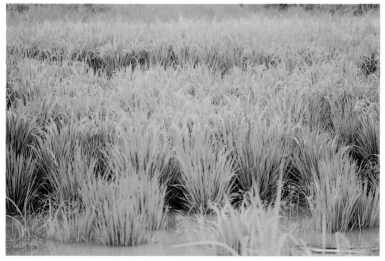

Fig. 152   Rice cultivated along the Napo River in northeast Peru.

Uses: Rice is probably the single most important crop in the world. Over 1.7 billion people are dependent on rice as a food staple. More than 200 million tons of it are consumed worldwide each year. Rice has been cultivated in Asia for more than 7,000 years, with its area of origin believed to be China or India. It is now grown throughout the world, including the southeastern and western United States. The major producer of upland rice is Brazil, which unfortunately has led to increased rainforest destruction to clear forest for rice fields. Throughout Latin America, rice and beans make up a significant and typical portion of most meals. In Amazonia, most subsistence farmers survive by growing and eating rice, plantains, and fish they catch in the rivers. The labor-intensive harvest by such people is always done by hand. The outer chaf is separated from the rice grains after the harvest in the Amazon by using a large mortar (*pilón*) and pestle (*mazo*). The *pilón*, a freestanding bowl-like receptacle carved from a single piece of wood, is filled with rice grains which are pounded with the *mazo*. The rice is scooped up and poured back periodically, allowing the chaf to float away from the grains.

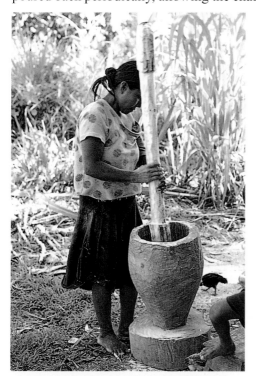

Fig. 153   Woman using a *pilón* (mortar) and *mazo* (pestle) to pound rice and separate the chaf from the grain (Amazonian Peru).

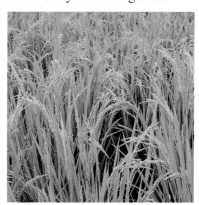

Fig. 154   Developing rice at a stage where the grains are still green.

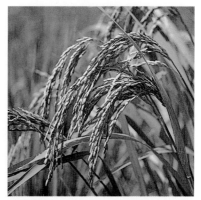

Fig. 155   Mature yellow-brown rice seedheads ready to be harvested.

Red Passion Vine
Granadilla Venenosa

Latin Name: *Passiflora coccinea* **Aubl.**
Passifloraceae: Passion Vine Family

Description: This climbing vine is also known as the red granadilla in English, although *granadilla* is the Spanish word for passion vine. The leaves are simple, alternate, and usually 3-lobed although sometimes lanceolate. They are approximately 7-10cm long and have a margin with regularly-spaced indentations that give the edge a slightly scalloped appearance. They are borne on short 2-3cm petioles. The distinctive flower is approximately 10cm in diameter and bright scarlet in color with yellowish pistils and stamens. It consists of ten red tepals (5 petals + 5 sepals) extending from the center. It is produced from an axillary bud on a stalk 7-10cm long. This vine climbs and attaches itself to supports by means of simple, twining, axillary tendrils. There are small cup-like structures (extra-floral nectaries) located on non-flower parts of the plant (especially the petiole apex / base of the leaf) that produce nectar and attract ants and wasps. These insects may benefit the plant by preying on other foliage-feeding insects present.

Uses: The AED states that both the fruit and flowers are edible, but the name *granadilla venenosa* (poison passion vine) indicates that at least some parts of the plant are poisonous. Cyanogenic compounds are known in this family (SAR). A brew of this plant is used to treat fever (VDF). A preparation from red passion vine is also used for conjunctivitis (GMJ).

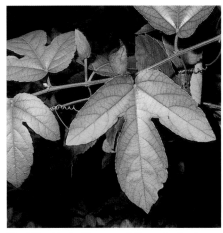
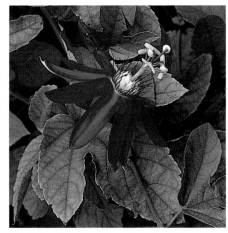

Fig. 156   Typical leaves and flower buds of the red passion vine.

Fig. 157   Flower of the red passion vine.

Purple Passion Vine
Maracuyá

Latin Name: *Passiflora edulis* Sims.
Passifloraceae: Passion Vine Family

Description: This is a climbing vine native to Brazil that is also known as the purple granadilla. It has simple, alternate leaves that are usually formed into three large finger-like lobes, each of which may come to a blunt point. The margins are slightly serrate. The mature leaves are roughly 10-12cm long by the same wide and show palmate venation with one main vein bisecting each lobe. They are borne on 3-5cm long petioles, each of which has two round cup-like glands (extra-floral nectaries) at its apex. This plant climbs by means of simple twining tendrils that emerge opposite a leaf and may have a dark or purplish color as new growth. A miniature cordate leaf-like structure (= stipule) is often present between the petiole and the stem. The purple and white flowers are 6-8cm in diameter, and are borne singly from the leaf axils. The flowers have ten tepals (five sepals, five petals), and five stamens, pigmented so there is a dark purple central area surrounded by lavender. The fruit is round to oval-shaped, about 8-10cm in diameter, and usually has a wrinkly leathery skin when mature. It starts out green, but becomes purple or red. Inside are many seeds surrounded by an aromatic yellow-orange pulp.

Uses: *Maracuyá* is known throughout Latin America as an edible fruit and a juice drink of the same name. The pulp is used in fruit salads and as a flavoring in sauces. It is heavily cultivated and exported. A brew from the leaves is used as a sedative, and the pure fruit juice as a heart tonic (AED).

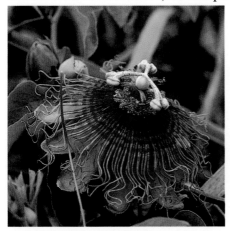

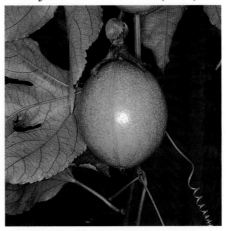

Fig. 158   The flower of the purple passion vine.   (Photo by Chris Campbell)

Fig. 159   The fruit of the purple passion vine.

Giant Granadilla
Tumbo

Latin Name: *Passiflora quadrangularis* L.
Passifloraceae: Passion Vine Family

Description: The giant granadilla has the typical characteristics shared by all species of *Passiflora* in being a climbing vine with simple , alternate leaves, simple tendrils used for support, and small cup-like glands (extra-floral nectaries) located on structures outside of the flower. It has large, broad, light green elliptical leaves that terminate in a short point and some-times reach a length of 25-30cm. Three pairs of large nectaries are found along the 5-8cm long petiole. The flowers are approximately 7-10cm in diameter with a predominantly purple color, although some parts are white, pink, and light green. The ovoid to ellipsoid fruit is large for a passion vine and may measure 20-25cm long by 10-15cm in diameter, and weigh 2-3kg. It is light green with a smooth surface and has three shallow longitudinal grooves. Within the fruit is a beige to dark green-colored fragrant pulp with a few scattered seeds. The stem of this plant is square, a character from which it derives its species name (quadrangularis = four-angled).

Uses: The giant granadilla is one of fifty edible species of passion fruit. As in the purple granadilla, the pulp and seeds are edible raw or can be used with the juice to make drinks or sorbets. Among the indigenous medical uses of the giant granadilla plant are: abortifacient (AED), treatment for bruises and fractures (RVM), treatment for inflammation, diabetes, arthritis, and hyper-tension (DAW). It is also used as a narcotic and sedative (DAW).

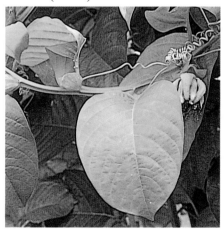

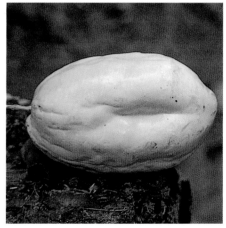

Fig. 160   Large entire leaf, tendrils, and opening flower of the giant granadilla.

Fig. 161   Fruit of the giant granadilla or *tumbo*.

Guarana
Guaraná

Latin Name: *Paullinia cupana* HBK. var. *sorbilis* (Mart.) Ducke
Sapindaceae: Soapberry Family

Description: Guarana is a woody vine or liana when it grows wild, but becomes a sprawling, climbing shrub when it is cultivated. It is indigenous to Brazil and found in the tropical forests of the Amazon Basin. It has alternate, compound leaves that are composed of one terminal leaflet and two pairs of opposite lateral leaflets. The leaflets are leathery, oval-elliptical with a short point, and dark green on the upper surface. They measure 15-30cm long by 10-15cm wide, and are borne on a winged rachis that is 15-20cm long. The inflorescence consists of small flowers in a cluster 15-30cm long. The fruit is a red to reddish-orange capsule that splits partially open along longitudinal membranes or grooves while still on the plant They are borne in large showy clusters and individually are approximately 2-3cm in diameter by 1-2cm thick. When open, they expose 1-3 round, dark brown seeds that are partially or almost completely covered with a white, mealy material (= aril) (CFNA).

Uses: The seeds of this plant have long been used by Amazonian Indians to prepare a drink or stimulant. The caffeine content of guarana is higher than that of coffee, tea, or cacao. Guarana is extremely popular in Brazil where it is marketed as powders, syrups, and soft drinks. In 1997, the Pepsi Co. released Josta in the U.S., a caffeine-rich soft drink derived from guarana. Preparations of the plant are taken for high blood pressure, headaches, dysentery, and fever (DAW, RAR). It is also considered an analgesic (MJB).

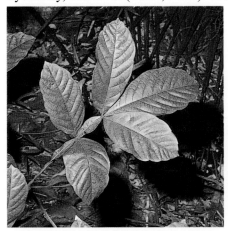

Fig. 162   Compound leaf of *guaraná*.

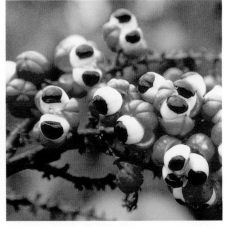

Fig. 163   Fruit of *guaraná*.
(Photo by Ghillean Prance)

Avocado
Palta, Aguacate

Latin Name: *Persea americana* Mill.
Lauraceae: Laurel Family

Description: Avocado is a medium-sized (15-20m) tree that is native to Central America and northwestern Amazonia. It has simple, entire, alternate leaves that are approximately 10-20cm long by 5-10cm wide. The leaves are oval to lanceolate in shape, usually coming to a distinct point but not extended into a drip-trip. The petioles are 2-5cm long. The leaves are dark green on top with an obvious yellow midvein and light green on the under surface where all the veins are prominent. The small green-white to green-yellow flowers are each less than a centimeter in diameter and borne in clusters at the ends of the branches. The fruits are typically 10-12cm long, dark green, and pear-shaped. The size and weight depends on the variety and may range from 250g to 1kg.

Uses: Avocado is cultivated throughout the tropics for its fruit which is rich in oil. Archaeological research indicates that it has been cultivated in Mexico for 9,000 years. It is eaten raw, often used in salads, and is the main component of guacamole. Extracts from the fruits, leaves, and seeds of avocado are used to treat a great variety of illnesses. Among its uses are as a contraceptive, as a snakebite treatment, and to clean the liver (SAR). Preparations are also used for anemia, diabetes, dysentery, and inflammation of the liver (RVM). Several sources mention its function as an aphrodisiac, which evidently was partially responsible for its original acceptance in the U.S.

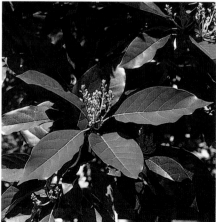

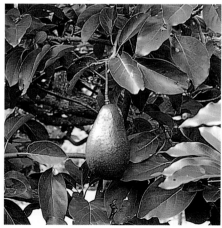

Fig. 164   Leaves and flowers of the avocado tree.

Fig. 165   Typical pear-shaped avocado fruit.

Garlic Weed
Mucura

Latin Name: *Petiveria alliacea* L.
Phytolaccaceae: Pokeweed Family

Description: This plant is a weedy herb that gets up to about a meter in height. It is found throughout the tropical areas of Central and South America. It gives off a garlic-like or onion-like smell if any of its parts are cut or crushed. The simple leaves are alternate and entire, elongate to lanceolate in shape, and come to a narrow point. The small white flowers are less than a centimeter long and are borne in widely-separated linear clusters on straight, upright spikes that are 20-40cm long. The longer stalks curve, but still usually remain well above the plant foliage. The small elongate fruits that develop contain one seed each and are dry and have bristles at the tip.

Uses: An extract of the root, well washed, cut up, and boiled in water is said to be taken during the first two months of pregnancy to cause an abortion (AMP). The leaves of this plant are used in magic rituals, and in therapeutic baths that are administered to give good feelings, increase thinking, and improve one's outlook on life (AMP). Bathing and washing with garlic weed-treated water is used for fevers and headaches (SAR). A preparation of the leaves is taken orally for lung ailments, while a liquid extract is used for earache (SAR). The AED cites many uses for this plant by indigenous tribes. Among the ailments it is used for are: rheumatism, cramps, beriberi, worms, scabies, arachnid stings and bites, paralysis, toothaches, and venereal disease (RAR). It may have curative properties against pancreatic cancer (JAD).

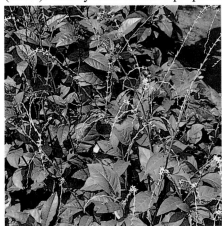

Fig. 166   Foliage and flower spikes of garlic weed.

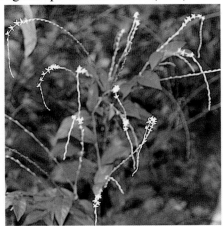

Fig. 167   Long flower spikes of garlic weed.

Stonebreaker
Chanca Piedra

Latin Name: *Phyllanthus niruri* L.
Euphorbiaceae: Spurge Family

Description: This plant is a small, low-growing herb seldom getting above half a meter in height. It is somewhat fern-like in appearance, especially when growing in dense concentrations. It has very small simple leaves that are alternately arranged on small branchlets of 5-10cm length. The foliage could easily be mistaken for a pinnately compound leaf. The tiny leaves are entire, ovate to obovate to elliptic, and come to a small point at the tip. The leaves are 8-10mm in length by about 2-3mm in width. The branchlets appear on the thin stem about every 3-5cm. The flowers are borne singly, one per leaf axil, beneath the branchlet. They are white and only 1-1.5mm in diameter. One green, pea-like fruit develops from the flower and also hangs beneath the branchlet on a short, thick stalk. The round fruit is approximately 2mm in diameter. A branchlet is very distinctive in profile due to the row of round green fruits hanging from the leaf axils and/or small white flowers. If present, flowers would be found towards the tip of the branchlet while the fruits would increase in size and stage of development as one approaches the stem . This genus lacks the white latex that is typical of other members of the family.

Uses: This plant is used to remove kidney stones and gall stones (NIC), and against viruses, bacteria, fever, and as a diuretic (TRA). It is also used as a pain reliever and to treat stomachache, constipation, diabetes, dysentery, flu, venereal problems, jaundice, malaria, and tumors (DAW).

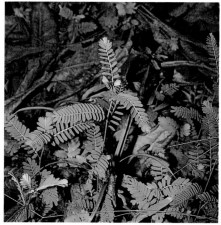

Fig. 168   The foliage of stonebreaker, consists of branchlets with many small, simple leaves.

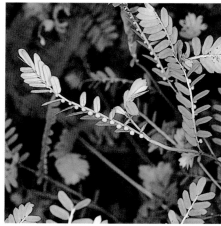

Fig. 169   Stonebreaker branchlet in profile showing the flowers near tip and hanging fruits.

Ivory Palm
Yarina, Tagua

Latin Name: ***Phytelephas aequatorialis*** **Spruce**
Arecaceae: Palm Family

Description: Ivory palm is the general term given to the six species of palms in this genus. The name itself, *Phytelephas*, comes from the Greek words meaning 'vegetable ivory', in reference to the hard white endosperm of the seeds. *P. aequatorialis* has a solitary trunk which attains a diameter of 30cm and a height of 15m. The long (2-3m) pinnate leaves are clustered at the top of the trunk and composed of 200-300 narrow, strap-like leaflets. The leaflets measure 40-50cm long by 3-5cm wide, being widest at their base and narrowing towards the tip. Dead leaves persist and may be present hanging from the trunk. Plants bear flowers of only one sex (= dioecious). The beige male flowers are borne in dense clusters on short stalks that radiate completely around a much larger and longer (.5-1m) central stalk. Fruits are produced in clusters of 3-8 with up to 20 per palm. The clusters are roundish and about 25-30cm in diameter. The woody, spiny fruits may be 12-15cm long by 7-10cm wide, and contain 4-6 seeds. *P. macrocarpa* has a subterranean stem and appears as a rosette of leaves from the ground with fruits at ground level.

Uses: *P. macrocarpa* is a diuretic (RAR). *P. aequatorialis* is the source of vegetable ivory or *tagua* that was exported commercially in the early 1900's from South America, primarily for button manufacture. It is used today for carvings and handicrafts. Leaf material has been used for roof thatch (AED), while the unripe fruit is consumed and considered a delicacy (HGB).

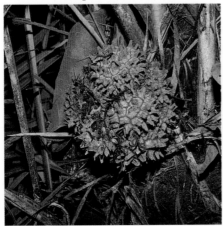

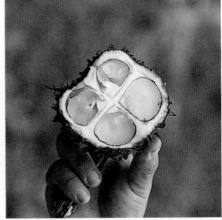

Fig. 170   A cluster of the spiny wooden fruits of an ivory palm.

Fig. 171   Fruit cross-section showing the white vegetable ivory or *tagua*.

Pokeberry
Jaboncillo

Latin Name: *Phytolacca rivinoides* **Kunth & Bouche**
Phytolaccaceae: Pokeweed Family

Description: This plant is a large herb that tends to become woody towards the base. It generally grows to 1-2m tall, but can get to be tree-like and grow to twice that size. It is distributed throughout Central America, northern South America, and the West Indies. The leaves are simple, alternate, elliptic to lance-shaped, with entire margins. The apex of the leaf may come to a long or short point. The leaves are typically 10-15cm long by 5-6cm wide, borne on petioles to 5cm in length. Small white flowers are borne on short stalks along both sides of a terminal or upper flower branch (= raceme) that may be 20-60cm in length and red to purple in color. The fruit is a rounded berry that is purplish-black, about .5cm in diameter, and very juicy at maturity.

Uses: This plant has been employed in some areas as a soap substitute for washing clothes, which has led to the Spanish common name provided above (*jabon* = soap) (SAR). Some Indian groups have used the leaves of pokeberry with those of plants in the genus *Phyllanthus* (page 98) to create a fish poison (SAR). The early shoots can be cooked as a vegetable (RAR). Indigenous uses also include preparations of the leaves to disinfect wounds and reduce their inflammation, as well as to decrease tumors (SAR). Pokeberry is sometimes used in a wash to treat rashes (AED).

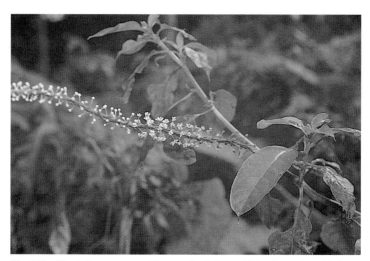

Fig. 172   The inflorescence and leaves of pokeberry (*Phytolacca rivinoides*).

Shoestring Pepper
Cordoncillo

Latin Name: *Piper* sp.
Piperaceae: Pepper Family

Description: This plant grows as a large bushy shrub to small tree 3-6m high. The large trunk is woody and about 10cm in diameter. It has simple, entire leaves that are alternately arranged in two ranks. Dark green above and light green below, the leaves are oval to lanceolate, but with an extremely long (5-7cm) drip-tip. Not counting the tips, the larger leaves range from 20-25cm long by 7-10cm wide. Secondary veins branch off diagonally from the midvein, but curve up towards the leaf tip before reaching the edge. The leaves emerge from a light green protective sheath such as seen in some figs. The terminal parts of the branches have dark green swollen nodal areas and light green hairy internodes, producing a bamboo-like appearance. Opposite each leaf is a single spicate flower stalk that is typical of the pepper family. These yellow to light green to white stalks are curved, arch-like, and very noticeable from a distance. If extended straight they would measure 12-18cm long.

Uses: The Spanish common name *cordoncillo* (which is applied to many species of *Piper*) means 'shoestring' and is derived from the long, slender spicate inflorescences. A mixture of the roots of this particular species in water is taken orally for kidney stones (AMP). It is also used for pains in the lower back and torso, and by women who have recently had babies to promote healing (AMP). This plant is also used to treat toothaches (JAD).

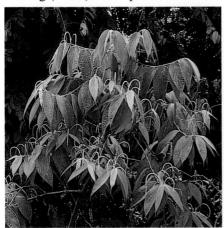

Fig. 173   The growth habit of *cordoncillo* (*Piper* sp.). Note the fruit and flower stalks.

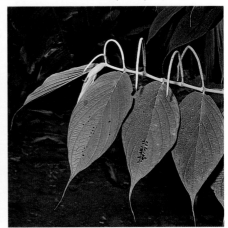

Fig. 174   The leaves and curving fruit and flower stalks of *cordoncillo* (*Piper* sp.).

Water Lettuce
Huama, Lechuga de Agua

Latin Name: *Pistia stratiotes* L.
Araceae: Arum or Aroid Family

Description: This plant is an atypical member of the aroid family, bearing little resemblance to the philodendrons or dieffenbachias that we know as ornamental plants and to which it is related. Water lettuce is a floating aquatic herb that grows in tropical areas worldwide. It is common in the Amazon, its tributaries, and in black water lakes. In some areas it grows in such dense populations that it covers the entire surface of the water. Water lettuce grows as a dense basal cluster of radiating leaves (= rosette), with usually free-floating roots dangling in the water. The leaves may be obovate to spatulate to almost rectangular in shape. The outer edge is rounded or may be notched (= emarginate). They are light green in color and have 6-8 parallel longitudinal grooves in their surface. Leaves range in size from 5-15cm long by 3-6cm wide, with usual plant diameters about 10-40cm. The inflorescences are small and not easily seen, occurring among the leaves. They consist of a very small dense spike (= spadix) of white flowers surrounded by a hood-like structure (= spathe). This plant is considered a weed in the U.S.

Uses: The crushed leaves of this plant have been used with salt to remove warts (SAR). Fungal diseases have been treated with the vapors from a leaf infusion of water lettuce (RVM).

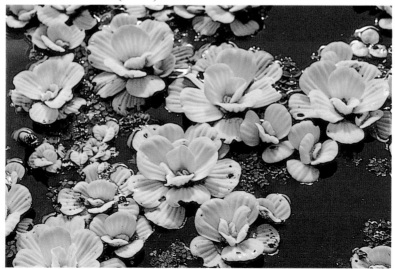

Fig. 175   Water lettuce (*Pistia stratiotes*) an aquatic floating herb

Frangipani
Suche Rosado

Latin Name: *Plumeria alba* L.
Apocynaceae: Dogbane Family

Description: Frangipani is a small tree usually found in dry forests ranging from 3-8m in height. Its branches are very fragile and tend to curve upwards, bearing large noticeable leaf scars. The leaves are simple and entire, alternate in arrangement, and clustered at the ends of the branches. They are oval in shape, come to a short point at the tip, and 20-40cm in length. There is a distinctive midvein with nearly perpendicular secondary veins which do not reach the leaf edge. The flower of *Plumeria alba* is white and approximately 5-8cm long with a narrow tubular base. The five petals flare out at the end with a diameter of 2-3cm. The flowers occur in small clusters. The fruits consist of dark brown, banana-shaped capsules that occur in opposite pairs arranged like a bull's horns. They range from 15-30cm in length and are borne on thick gray stalks that are sometimes branched to carry several pairs of fruits, attaching in the center of each pair of capsules. They dry out and split open to reveal large (3-4cm) wind-dispersed seeds that resemble those of pine cones with a large single asymmetrical wing. This plant produces a milky latex.

Uses: Frangipani is widely cultivated as an ornamental tree. Medicinally, it has been used as a stimulant, heart tonic, and purgative (DAW). It is poisonous and kills some bacteria and fungi (DAW). Preparations have been used to treat rheumatism, venereal disease, tumors, fever, and skin problems (DAW).

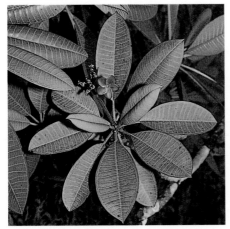

Fig. 176 *Plumeria alba* varies from *P. rubra* (shown here) only in having white flowers.

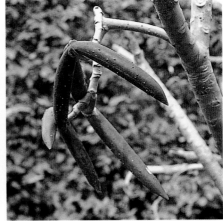

Fig. 177   The fruit pods of *Plumeria alba*.

Purslane
Verdolaga

Latin Name: *Portulaca oleracea* L.
Portulacaceae: Purslane Family

Description: Purslane is native to northern Africa, but can now be found worldwide. It is a fleshy or succulent annual herb that grows very close to the ground (= prostrate). It generally grows in radial fashion, spreading out from the center, but may also exhibit a creeping growth form. It is commonly found in disturbed sites. Purslane has alternate, entire, elliptic to inversely egg-shaped (= obovate) succulent leaves that are 1-3cm long by .5-1cm wide (TBC). The leaves are borne on short petioles that are less than a centimeter long and may not be noticeable. The small yellow flowers have four petals and are clustered near the ends of the stems. Flowers are usually small and may attain one centimeter in diameter. The fruits are nearly round capsules 2-3mm in diameter. The seeds within are black and minute, approximately one millimeter in diameter. Purslane may get up to 40cm long, but is more commonly less than half that length.

Uses: The stems and leaves of purslane are used to increase urine flow and relieve headaches, or when applied in poultice form to treat wounds and sores, heal ulcers, and stop bleeding (AAB). The crushed plant is used to treat bee stings, fever, and swellings (AED). Leaves and stems can be boiled and eaten (AAB). The AED lists a wide range of recorded uses and sicknesses that can be treated with purslane. A selection of these are: sedative, fungicide, vermifuge, and gonorrhea, hepatitis, dysentery, herpes, and boils.

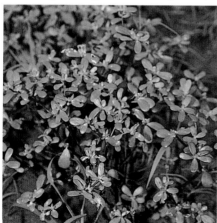

Fig. 178　Purslane, a low-growing succulent herb.

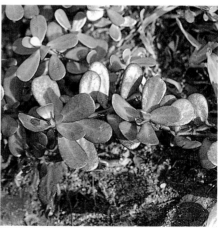

Fig. 179　Close-up of the small succulent leaves of purslane.

Snake Bite Plant
Curarina

Latin Name: *Potalia amara* Aubl.
Loganiaceae: Logania Family

Description: Snake bite plant is indigenous to the lowland tropical forests of South America and is found commonly throughout the Amazon Basin, especially on nutrient deficient soils. It is the single species found within the genus *Potalia*, and is sometimes even elevated to the rank of its own family (the Potaliaceae). It is an understory treelet whose leaves grow clustered together at the top of the stem or small trunk (= pachycaul). The cultivated specimen examined was approximately one meter tall. This plant has large, opposite, entire, stiff leathery leaves. These leaves are long and narrow with an oblanceolate shape (= wider towards the tip). The leaves terminate in a short point. Typical mature leaves are 25-35cm long by 8-12cm wide (at their widest point). The leaves narrow towards the base into a short, thickened, laterally-flattened petiole. The flowers are borne in clusters at the top of the stem and give rise to round fruits.

Uses: Snake bite plant is a name 'coined' by the authors due to the widespread reports in the literature of its usage in varying preparations for this purpose. The mottled patterning on the trunk of the plant suggests a Doctrine of Signatures usage (SAR). Some of the other uses of this plant are as an analgesic and to treat opthalmia, poisoning, venomous ant stings, and the sting from the fresh-water skate (SAR). Snake bite plant is also used to treat venereal diseases (AED) and to promote the healing of cavities (RVM).

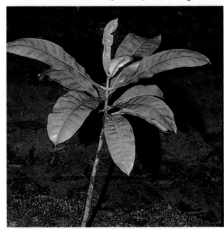

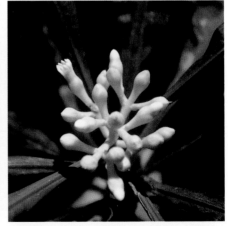

Fig. 180   Typical growth form of the snake bite plant with leaves clustered at top of stem.

Fig. 181   A cluster of flowers of the snake bite plant .   (Photo by Ghillean Prance)

Guava
Guayaba

Latin Name: *Psidium guajava* L.
Myrtaceae: Myrtle Family

Description: Guava is a shrub to small tree that typically grows from 5-10m in height. It is native to Brazil, but is now cultivated throughout the tropical areas of the world. It is a common tree in secondary growth. The leaves are simple, entire, and opposite in arrangement. They are oval to elliptic in shape and rounded at the tip or come to a very small point. They range from about 8-12cm long by 3-6cm wide and are borne on short petioles of approximately one centimeter. The flowers have five white petals, many stamens, and are found solitary in the leaf axils. They are 3-4cm in diameter. The large berries are round to somewhat pear-shaped, green when young turning yellow with maturity, and approximately 4-6cm in diameter. The flesh inside is pink and contains many seeds.

Uses: Guava is cultivated as an ornamental and its fruit is highly prized for its taste. It has a higher Vitamin C content than citrus fruits, and is also high in Vitamin A (SWPT). The leaves are chewed for mouth sores and the bark is employed to relieve dysentery (ESG, SWPT). Preparations of the flowers are used to help regulate menstrual periods (FOR). Other uses of guava include treating emotional shock, vertigo, bleeding gums, itching, vomiting, hang-overs, and for relaxing the vagina following childbirth (AED, SWPT, AAB). A related species, *Psidium acutangulum*, is used as an astringent (SAR).

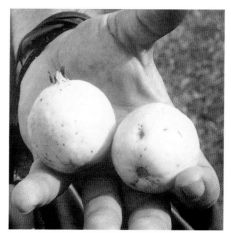

Fig. 182   Ripe guava fruits.

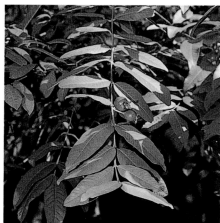

Fig. 183   Leaves and developing fruits of the guava tree.

Psychotria
Yagé

Latin Name: *Psychotria* spp.
Rubiaceae: Madder or Coffee Family

Description: There are over 700 species of *Psychotria* found in the New World, many of which are common throughout the Amazon Basin. These plants are shrubs to small trees that have simple, opposite, entire leaves. The flowers are usually white or yellow, occurring in terminal spikes. The fruits are roundish berries that become red or purplish at maturity. The following description applies to a species that was identified only as *yagé* in Peru. This plant is bush-like, 2-3m in height. The leaves are 10-20cm long by 5-7cm wide, smooth and shiny, and slightly wavy or wrinkled in appearance. They are lanceolate to ovate. Small white flowers are borne in a cluster on a 7-10cm long spike that arises at the tips of the branches. The individual flowers are tubular and measure approximately 1cm long by .5cm in diameter.

Uses: The species of *Psychotria* referred to as *yagé* are used by the Indians of Amazonia as an additive to the preparation of the hallucinogenic drink *ayahuasca*. This drink (page 8) is also called *yagé*, as is the liana called soul vine (*Banisteriopsis caapi*, page 21) which makes up its primary ingredient. The addition of *Psychotria* material greatly heightens the effect of the drug. Additional uses include the root of *P. acuminata* in a treatment for children who urinate too frequently (AED). The leaves of *P. deflexa* are used in bath water to relieve fever in children (FOR), and in *P. poepiggiana* as an analgesic.

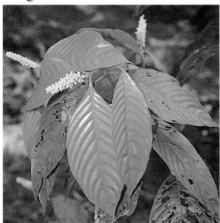

Fig. 184   Leaves and inflorescences of *Psychotria* sp. identified as *yagé*.

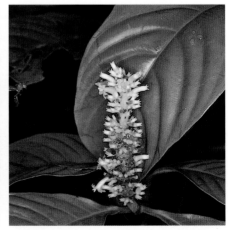

Fig. 185   Inflorescence of *Psychotria* sp. identified as *yagé*.

Dwarf Ginger
Mishquipanga Enano

Latin Name: *Renealmia alpinia* (Rottb.) Maas
Zingiberaceae: Ginger Family

Description: This species of ginger seldom gets beyond a meter in height (AMP), hence the Spanish common name (*enano* = dwarf) and the English common name 'coined' by the authors. Dwarf ginger grows as a cluster of reddish-tinted stems of 1-2cm diameter, bearing alternate, entire, lanceolate leaves. Unlike gingers in the genus *Costus* (pages 42-43), the leaves of dwarf ginger are thin rather than fleshy and have an open rather than clasping leaf sheath. There is a distinct yellow midvein and secondary veins are slightly depressed forming shallow diagonal grooves in the leaf surface. The pointed leaves emerge in a tight roll and can reach a size of 30-45cm long by 12-15cm wide. The flowers are red, 2-3cm long, and are produced in clusters on a stalk composed of loosely overlapping bracts. These inflorescences are usually close to the base of the plant, ranging from 5-40cm high. The fruits are elliptical red capsules to 3cm in length (TBC).

Uses: This species might also be nicknamed 'dye ginger' since both the roots and the fruits are used by different native groups in extracting dyes. A yellow to reddish-orange one is produced from the root, while a red-purple to black dye is produced from the fruits (SAR) and used on fabrics and handicrafts (AED). Medicinally, the leaves are used in baths for people who are especially nervous or sad (AMP). Also used in some way to help divine where animals are in the forest when one needs to hunt (AMP).

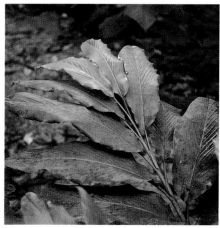

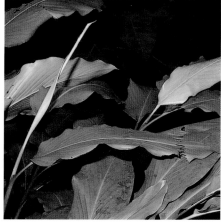

Fig. 186   Leaves of the dwarf ginger
(*Renealmia alpinia*).

Fig. 187   Tightly curled new growth of the
dwarf ginger (*Renealmia alpinia*).

Castor Bean
Higuerilla

Latin Name: *Ricinus communis* L.
Euphorbiaceae: Spurge Family

Description: The castor bean plant is usually seen as an upright weedy shrub 2-3m in height, but can grow to be a small tree attaining a height of ten meters in the tropics. It is believed indigenous to Africa, but has been introduced and established throughout the New World (SAO). The large leaves are simple and palmate, containing 4-9 finger-like lobes that have serrate margins. The venation is palmate, with one main vein bisecting each lobe. Leaves range in diameter from 15-45cm and are borne on long (10-30cm) petioles that attach to the bottom surface well within the edge of the leaf (= peltate). New growth is often red or dark. The flowers occur in spike-like inflorescences 10-30cm long, with hairy maroon-red female flowers on top and smaller white male flowers below. The fruits are spiny, 3-lobed, brown capsules about 2-3cm in length. Each yields three brown or mottled seeds.

Uses: The seeds (castor 'beans') are pressed to extract the oil which makes up more than half their weight. Castor oil was once commonly used as a laxative and often given to children. The seeds, hulls, and unrefined oil however are extremely toxic. Castor bean is cultivated commercially for oil production primarily in India and China, and to a much lesser degree in Brazil and Paraguay. The oil today is used mainly in soaps, paints, and as a lubricant in airplane engines (SAO). In traditional medicine, the leaves are used to reduce fevers, and to help heal cuts, sores, swellings, and headaches (AAB).

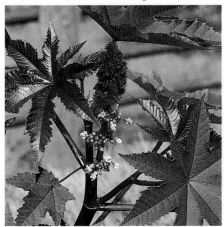

Fig. 188   Red female flowers and white male flowers of the castor bean plant.

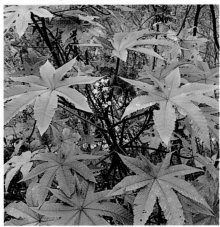

Fig. 189   Foliage and flowers of the castor bean plant (*Ricinus communis*).

Sugar Cane
Caña de Azúcar

Latin Name: *Saccharum officinarum* L.
Poaceae: Grass Family

Description: Sugar cane belongs to the grass family, which includes rice and the other cereal grains. Sugar cane is a thick-stemmed perennial grass with long pointed narrow leaves that are distributed regularly in alternate fashion along the stem. The leaves may reach a length of 3-4m, and resemble a giant blade of grass. The sugar cane stem is jointed, and the leaf sheath clasps the stem where they meet. There is usually a dark ring of discoloration at the nodes which gives the stem a bamboo-like appearance. The venation in the leaves is parallel. The flowers are reduced and adapted for wind pollination. They are borne on a tall stalk in pyramid-shaped clusters that rise above the plant. The cane itself may reach a height of 6-8m. Because of the dense, closely-packed manner in which the stems grow, sugar cane sometimes has a weedy appearance and may be mistaken for other grasses or rushes such as *caña brava* (*Gynerium sagittatum*) that grow along the riverbanks in Amazonia.

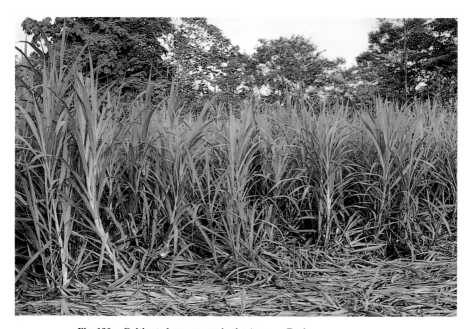

Fig. 190   Cultivated sugar cane in the Amazon Basin.

Uses: Sugar cane is grown to make and refine sugar, which is processed from the juice that collects in the pith of the stem. The only strict medicinal use of sugar cane found was a treatment involving the warm sap which is used for infected eyes (SAR). Today, sugar cane is cultivated throughout the tropical areas of the world, but is believed to have originated in New Guinea and been dispersed by means of human migration. Sugar cane is often stripped and eaten or sucked raw by indigenous people where it is grown. Sugar cane and its by-products have several other uses. In Amazonia, the sugar cane juice is extracted and then fermented into a liquor called *aguardiente*. The juice may also be boiled down into a thick dark molasses, sometimes in large copper bowls or cauldrons. The crushed, flattened cane stem (= bagasse) that remains after juice extraction has been used in different countries to make paper, chipboard, and as cattle food. Fermented sugar cane stems and leaves are currently being used as the main ingredients of 'gasohol', an alcohol-based fuel for running specially engineered vehicles. A quarter of the cars now made in Brazil run on gasohol.

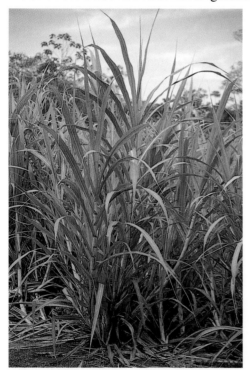

Fig. 191   A single clump of sugar cane plants.

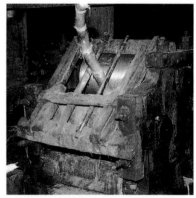

Fig. 192   Sugar cane stalk entering press to extract the juice.

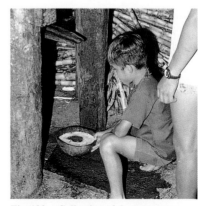

Fig. 193   Collection of the raw sugar cane juice as cane is being pressed.

Sweet Broom
Ñucñupichana

Latin Name: *Scoparia dulcis* L.
Scrophulariaceae: Foxglove Family

Description: This plant is a small, low-growing herbaceous weed that is common in the tropical lowlands. Portions of its names in English, Spanish, Quechua, and Latin mean 'sweet', but no reference could be found to a sweet fragrance or taste associated with this species. The narrow stems are angular in appearance due to longitudinal ribs running their length. The small leaves are opposite and oblanceolate in shape, narrowing at the base but without an obvious petiole. The margins are entire with the apical half toothed. They are approximately 1.5-2cm long by .5cm wide, with usually two or three at a node. There are multiple side branches which grow diagonally from the main branches resulting in a geometrical appearance to the foliage. Most lateral branches occur in opposite pairs. The flowers are very small, white or tinged with lavender. Clusters of several buds emerge from the leaf axils at the nodes and are borne on stalks 2-3 times their length.

Uses: Amazonian Indians use this plant to treat aches and pains, swellings, wounds, and as a contraceptive (SAR). In the latter case, sweet broom may be mixed with *Chenopodium ambrosioides* (page 35). Leaves of the plant are often tied together to fashion a makeshift broom commonly used (hence the name)(RVM). The juice of the leaf is used to treat eye problems (BDS). Preparations are also used to treat bronchitis and coughs, dysentery, kidney ailments, fever, and hemorrhoids (RVM, VDF).

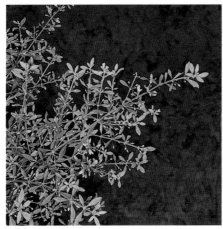

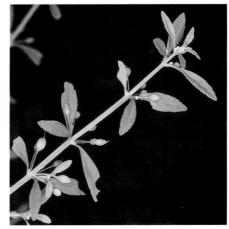

Fig. 194   The geometrically-branching foliage of sweet broom.

Fig. 195   Close-up of the leaves and flower buds of sweet broom.

Spike Moss
Shapumba

Latin Name: *Selaginella* spp.
Selaginellaceae: Spike Moss Family

Description: *Selaginella* is the only genus of the spike moss family. It consists of more than 500 species of small to medium-sized plants found in tropical rainforests. Their growth habit may be erect, climbing, or very low to the point of becoming a ground cover with dense populations. The scale-like leaves are generally of two different shapes (= dimorphic). Leaves are typically less than a centimeter long and have a single vein. The leaves usually grow in a single plane giving the plant a flattened appearance. Its branching and color usually impart it a feathery, fern-like appearance as well. Spike mosses are not seed-bearing plants and produce only spores from small cone-like reproductive structures (= strobili). The spike mosses in the Amazon Basin tend to grow low and sprawl over the ground.

Uses: In some areas, a tea is made from boiling the roots for problems of the pancreas and stomach (*S. exaltata* and *S. speciosa*) (FOR). A decoction of the plant is used as a bath for treating influenza (*S. stellata*) (BDS). These plants are sometimes picked for ornamental or decorative purposes (AED).

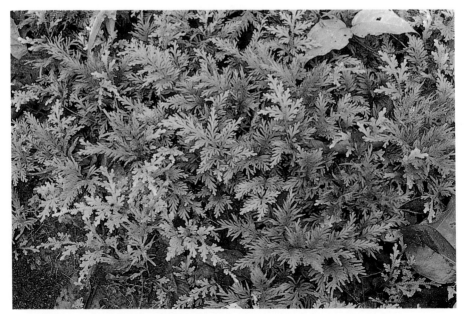

Fig. 196   A bed of fern-like spike moss (*Selaginella* sp.) growing along the forest floor.

Wild Senna
Retama Amarilla

Latin Name: *Senna reticulata* (Willd.) H. Irwin & Barneby
Caesalpiniaceae: Caesalpinia Family

Description: Wild senna is a small tree or large shrub that is often found along the edges of streams and can reach a height of 6-8 meters. The leaves are even pinnately compound and usually have from 12-20 ovate to obovate leaflets that increase in size from the base of the leaf to the tip. A mature leaf may be 30-50cm long by 12-20cm wide, and is borne on a petiole that is swollen at its base (= pulvinus). Bright yellow flowers occur in terminal spikes giving rise to the Spanish common name of *retama amarilla* (= yellow broom). Each flower has five petals and is about 3-4cm across. Flowers at the bottom of the spike open first. The fruits are flattened pods that are green and curvy initially, but dark and straight at maturity, attaining a length of 15 centimeters.

Uses: This plant is often cultivated as an ornamental due to its showy flowers, but also has a variety of medicinal uses. The flowers are used to treat liver problems as well as upset stomachs (AED). Both the leaves and the flowers contain antibiotics that are effective against certain bacteria and useful in treating kidney inflammations (AED). Wild senna is also used to treat venereal and skin problems (RVM) and as a medication against ring-worm (AED). The leaves are sometimes used as an insect repellent by some indigenous groups, while others use the plant against fungal infections (SAR).

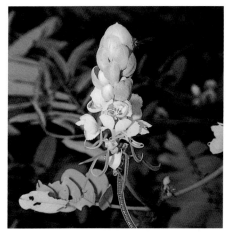

Fig. 197   A cluster of the flowers of wild senna with developing fruit pods.

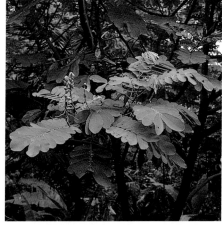

Fig. 198   The pinnately compound leaves and yellow blossoms of wild senna.

Simarouba
Marupá

Latin Name: ***Simarouba amara*** **Aubl.**
Simaroubaceae: Simarouba Family

Description: This is a small genus with only five species, all of which are canopy trees that have alternate pinnately compound leaves and a bitter-tasting bark. The following description is based on a specimen three meters in height that was observed in cultivation. The leaves are extremely long, ranging from 45-90cm and have an even number of leaflets (24-42). The leaflets are thick and leathery, with almost a rubbery texture and appearance. Individual leaflets have parallel margins and are rounded at the tip or with a short point, ranging in size from 7-12cm long by 3-5cm wide. The petiolule is about a centimeter long. Leaflets do not form along the leaf rachis for a distance of 15-20cm from the trunk. The following is based on information from Croat (TBC). The small green flowers are less than a centimeter long and occur in 30cm long clusters (= panicles) at the ends of the branches. The small fruits are oval-shaped and about 1.5-2cm long. They are green while young, turning red-orange to black. Height ranges from 5-35 meters.

Uses: The bark of *S. amara* is chopped up and boiled in water, which is then taken orally to treat high fever (AMP). This treatment results in frequent diarrhea. In some areas the bark is taken with rum as a treatment for malaria and dysentery (GMJ). Other recorded uses include a purgative and emetic, and to staunch blood flow (RAR). This species has been used for a variety of commercial lumber applications (AED).

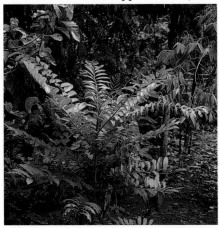

Fig. 199   Foliage of a young *Simarouba amara* tree.

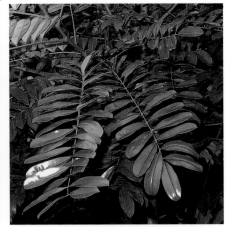

Fig. 200   Close-up showing the compound leaves of a *Simarouba amara* tree.

Siparuna
Picho Huayo

Latin Name: *Siparuna guianensis* Aubl.
Monimiaceae: Monimia Family

Description: This plant is a shrub or small tree, seldom exceeding five meters in height. It has wide, leathery leaves that narrow at both ends and come to a point at the tip. The leaves are opposite, simple, and entire and usually occur 2-3 at a node. They range in size from 35-45cm long by 15-20cm wide (at their widest central point). The leaves are borne on 1-3cm long petioles and have diagonal secondary veins that curve up towards the leaf tip as they approach the margin. The small greenish inconspicuous flowers occur in small clusters in the leaf axils on either side of the stem. They develop into distinctive, reddish, fig-like fruits which eventually split open to reveal a pink interior with a shiny red seed. The top-shaped unopen fruits are about 2-3cm long by the same in diameter. Once open, they may be star-shaped and resemble a flower blossom. This plant has a pungent vegetative odor.

Uses: The fruits are consumed by one Indian group as a remedy for indigestion (SAR). Preparations of the leaves are used to treat a variety of ills. In baths as a treatment for fungal infections, while as a tea for accelerating the delivery of a baby, alleviating a fever, and to induce an abortion (AED). The odor of the crushed leaves rubbed over the body is used to mask the odor of hunters from the game they seek, and also purportedly has the effect of an aphrodisiac (JAD). Additionally, this plant has been used in traditional medicine for colds, cramps, skin infections, rheumatism, and wounds (DAW).

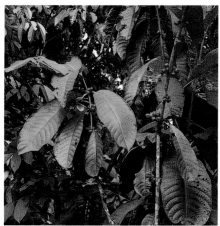

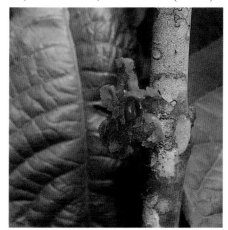

Fig. 201   Foliage and clusters of unopened fruits of *Siparuna guianensis*.

Fig. 202   Close-up of the opened fruit with seed of *Siparuna guianensis*.

Stilt Palm
Pona

Latin Name: *Socratea exorrhiza* (Mart.) H.Wendl.
Arecaceae: Palm Family

Description: These palms are found throughout Central and northern South America in tropical forests below 1000m elevation. They typically range from 10-20m in height and 15-18cm diameter. Although similar to *Iriartea deltoidea*, *Socratea* differs by having stilt roots which are densely covered with spines and that form a 'root cone' that one can see through. There are usually 6-8 long pinnate leaves whose sheaths form a smooth green slightly swollen crownshaft at the top of the trunk. Often a new leaf is seen sticking straight up from the center of the crown. The leaflets are wider and ragged at the apex, and split into segments. When in flower, thickly-packed small white blossoms along 30-40cm long branches hang down at the base of the crownshaft. The yellow oval fruit are 3-4cm long by 2-3cm in diameter.

Uses: Bark from the trunk is split off and used as flooring slats, walls, and dividers (AED). The spiny stilt roots are used as graters (HGB). Different tribes use a leaf brew or the roots as treatment for hepatitis (AYA, NIC).

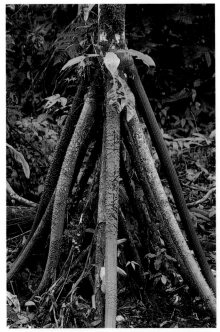

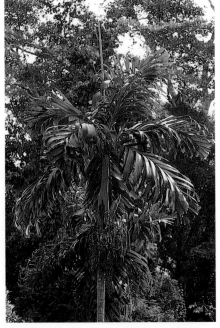

Fig. 203 *Socratea exorrhiza* forms a root cone of spiny stilt roots that you can see through.

Fig. 204 The leaves, crownshaft, and flower branches of the stilt palm *Socratea exorrhiza*.

Breast Berry
Cocona Venenosa

Latin Name: *Solanum mammosum* L.
Solanaceae: Nightshade or Potato Family

Description: This plant grows as a low shrub or herb, usually about 1-2m in height. The broad leaves are simple and alternate, with margins that have broad angular lobes. Several large spines may protrude from the upper and lower leaf surfaces along the veins. They are reminiscent in size and shape to the leaves of many varieties of eggplant, which belong to the same genus. The medium-sized open star-shaped flowers occur in small clusters. The breast berry bush is so named because of the yellow-orange fruits which are adorned with multiple breast-like protuberances. These irregularly-shaped fruits are about 10-15cm long and 8-10cm in diameter. The individual breast-shaped protuberances on the fruit are typically 3-5cm long by 2-3cm in diameter.

Uses: The fruits of the breast berry plant are evidently poisonous, which would explain the Spanish common name of *cocona venenosa* (= poisonous cocona). Multiple sources list several different Indian tribes as using the fruit and/or seeds as an insecticide, specifically to kill cockroaches (SAR, FOR, CAA). Given the previous usage, it seems strange that the fruits are also evidently employed as pacifiers (SAR). One indigenous group uses the fruit mashed up in hot water to treat growths of the breast, suggesting an obvious Doctrine of Signatures usage (AED). The fruit juice is used in preparations to treat asthma, arthritis, and rheumatism (POV). Fruit are also used to treat the ulcers caused by leishmaniasis (DAT).

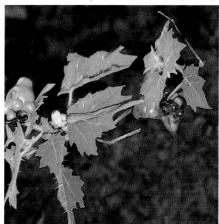

Fig. 205   The breast berry bush has large spiny leaves with shallow angular lobes.

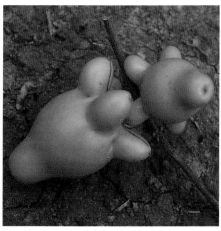

Fig. 206   The fruit of the breast berry bush has numerous swellings for which it is named.

Tree Tomato
Gallinazo Panga

Latin Name: *Solanum obliquum* R. & P.
Solanaceae: Nightshade or Potato Family

Description: Tree tomato grows as a shrub to small tree about 2-5 meters tall. It has a straggly, upright growth form with the older growth woody and the younger green, smooth, and soft-wooded. The leaves are simple, alternate, and slightly asymmetrical. They have entire margins and are usually pointed, with the shape ranging from ovate to cordate. Young or juvenile leaves may be deeply lobed. Mature leaves are usually 8-20cm long by 6-15cm wide, borne on petioles of 3-8cm in length. The leaves have a distinctive foul odor when crushed. The star-shaped flowers are approximately 2-3cm across, have five light green petals with brown or purple markings, and five erect yellow to white stamens that surround a central green pistil. The round green flower buds develop uniquely, uncurling from a pendent stalk with the youngest in the center of the curl which may hold 10-20 buds. The pendent fruits may be single or in clusters, turning from green to yellow when mature. The fruits are round to oval in shape and 3-5cm long, hanging from pendent stalks at branch forks. Tree tomato was formerly placed in the genus *Cyphomandra*, and is listed under that name in older publications (and as *C. hartwegii* in the AED).

Uses: The fruits of this tree are edible. Sometimes they are squeezed to obtain the juice which is then used for painting ceramics and pottery (SAR). One Indian group uses a 'bath' made from this tree in an effort to protect babies from a weakness based on one of their superstitions (AED).

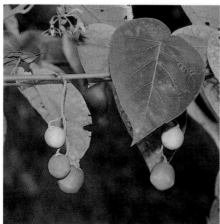

Fig. 207   Leaves and pendent fruits of tree tomato.

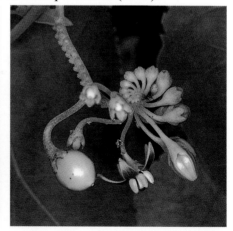

Fig. 208   A flower, buds, and young developing fruit of the tree tomato.

Cocona
Cocona

Latin Name: *Solanum sessiliflorum* **Dun.**
Solanaceae: Nightshade or Potato Family

Description: Cocona is very similar in growth habit and appearance to breast berry (*Solanum mammosum*, page 118), which is in the same genus. This low shrub seldom gets over two meters high and is often laden with fruit found in clusters on its branches. The leaves look like oversized eggplant leaves, with several to a dozen shallow teeth or points along the margin. The leaves are alternate, simple, and widely spaced along the stem. They have a distinctive yellow midvein and several obvious secondary veins that diverge from it to the leaf's margin. The leaves may be very large, sometimes reaching a length of 45cm and a width of 30cm. They are borne on petioles of 5-10cm length. Flowers are typical of *Solanum*, star-shaped, containing five petals and anthers, and in cocona about 3cm in diameter. A relative of the tomato, the fruits are about 3-5cm in diameter, round, and green initially but developing to yellow or orange at maturity.

Uses: Cocona is grown throughout the Amazon Basin. Juice squeezed from the fruit is high in Vitamin C and often used as a drink. Some indigenous people crush the leaves to extract a liquid that is used as a treatment for burns, to alleviate pain and avoid blistering and scarring (AMP). The juice is taken orally and used topically to avoid vomiting and heal dead tissue, respectively, following envenomizations by arachnids (SAR), and snakebites (RVM). Juice is also used as a scalp treatment, cosmetically and medically (SAR).

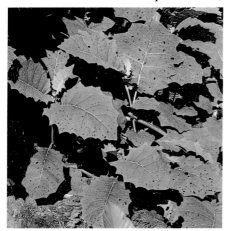

Fig. 209 Cocona grows as a small shrub or bush throughout the Amazon Basin.

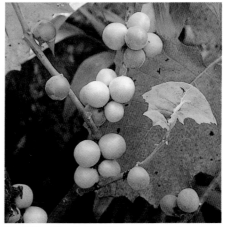

Fig. 210 The fruits of the cocona are tomato-sized, and turn orange as they mature.

Strychnine
Comida del Venado

Latin Name: *Strychnos guianensis* (Aubl.) C. Mart.
Loganiaceae: Logania Family

Description: The genus *Strychnos* has dozens of species that are indigenous to the tropical forests of the Amazon Basin, most of which grow as climbing shrubs or thick lianas. They are easily recognized due to their characteristic leaf venation. They have three obvious longitudinal veins (one on either side of the midvein) that all originate from the same point near the base of the leaf. The only other neotropical plant families with 3-veined leaves are the Melostomataceae and the Buxaceae. *S. guianensis* is one of the most common species in the Amazon region. It has simple, narrowly ovate, opposite leaves that come to a point. The small tubular flowers each have five petals and occur in clusters in the leaf axils. The fruits of this vine are rounded capsules.

Uses: This species has been used to treat venereal diseases by mixing it with *Uncaria guianensis* (page 126) and bathing the infected area. However, the most widespread indigenous use of this plant and other species of *Strychnos* in the Amazon is as an ingredient in the preparation of the arrow-poison curare. The bark of at least 12 species has been recorded used for this purpose (SAR), and may serve either as the primary constituent or as an additive when used with other plants such as *Chondrodendron tomentosum* (page 36). Plants in the genus *Strychnos* are rich in alkaloids, which are usually most heavily concentrated in the bark. Among them are strychnine and tubocurarine, the latter still used in Western medicine as a muscle relaxant during anesthesia.

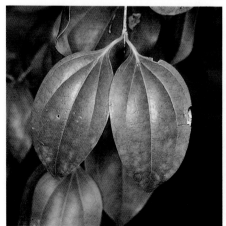

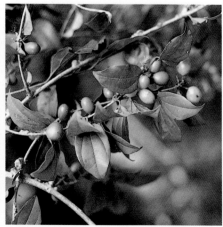

Fig. 211 Characteristic 3-veined opposite leaves of strychnos (*Strychnos spinosa*).

Fig. 212 Vine of *Strychnos* sp. with fruits. (Photo by Ghillean Prance)

Cocoa or Chocolate Tree
Cacao

Latin Name: *Theobroma cacao* L.
Sterculiaceae: Sterculia or Cacao Family

Description: The cocoa tree is found under natural conditions in the primary forests of the Orinoco and Upper Amazon River Basins where it can reach a height of 12-16 meters. Under open plantation or the orchard conditions of cultivation, the tree is usually no more than 5-6m high. The large leathery leaves are simple, have entire margins, and are alternately arranged. They are oval to oblong in shape, coming to a short but distinctive point. They range from 15-50cm long by 4-10cm wide, and are borne on petioles that vary greatly in length (2-10cm) and that are swollen at both ends. The secondary veins alternate in diagonal fashion from the midvein, but curve up towards the point before reaching the margin and actually merge into the next secondary vein. The small uniquely-shaped flowers are borne on the branches and trunk (= cauliflory) usually in clusters of 10-25. The petals are white to pink with some maroon coloration that matches the filaments protruding from the center. The blossoms are 1-1.5cm in diameter and borne on stems of 1-3cm length. The fruit is a thick-skinned oval capsule, green to yellow to red in color, that contains up to 20-60 seeds surrounded by an aromatic edible white pulp. They grow up to 15-20cm long by 6-12cm wide from a short thick stalk, and have ten longitudinal grooves in their smooth surface.

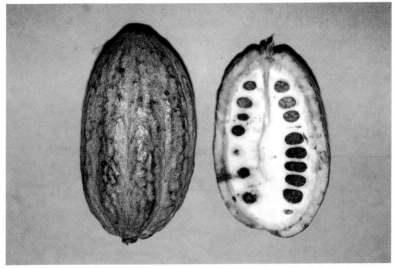

Fig. 213   A mature cacao pod opened to show the white pulp and dark 'beans'.

Uses: Cacao is a commercially important product consumed throughout the world in both liquid (cocoa) and solid (chocolate) forms. Historical records indicate that cocoa was used in pre-Columbian times by Indian groups such as the Maya, Aztecs, and Zapotecs. Traditional preparation of cocoa starts with removing the beans or seeds from the pod, roasting them, shelling them, and then grinding the inner seed to produce a chocolate powder. The white pulp that surrounds the seeds is also sweet and edible. The adaptive basis for this is to attract wild animals that carry off the pods and serve as seed dispersers. Extracts of the leaves are used by indigenous tribes as a heart tonic and as a diuretic (SAR). Brews from the bark and the toasted seeds are used to treat other ailments (SAR). Certain chemical extracts are currently used as asthma treatments (JAD). Cocoa butter is widely used in suppositories (AED). The name *Theobroma* translates as 'food of the gods'. The largest cacao producers are the Ivory Coast, Brazil, and Malaysia. Cocoa (the chocolate drink) and the cacao tree should not be confused with *coca* (= cocaine in Spanish, see *Erythroxylon coca* page 52), nor with *coco* (= coconut in Spanish).

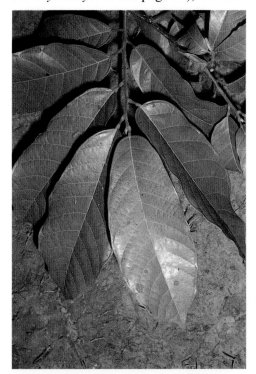

Fig. 214   Leaves of the cocoa or chocolate tree (*Theobroma cacao*).

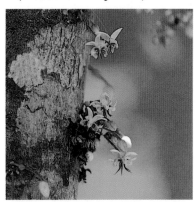

Fig. 215   Cocoa tree blossoms may emerge from a branch or directly from the trunk.

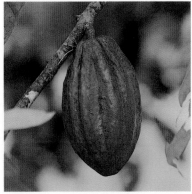

Fig. 216   A mature fruit pod of the cocoa tree.

Yellow Oleander
Camalonga

Latin Name: *Thevetia peruviana* (Pers.) Schumann
Apocynaceae: Dogbane Family

Description: Yellow oleander is also called 'lucky nut' or 'be-still tree' in English, and *bellaquillo* or *flor amarilla* in Spanish. It is a large shrub or small tree that is indigenous to the mountain valleys of the Andes. It is characterized by the typical milky white sap usually found in this family of plants. *T. peruviana* has very distinctive long linear leaves that resemble those of the ornamental oleander (*Nerium oleander*) often used as a landscape plant in warmer areas of the United States, and from which it takes one of its English common names. Theses linear leaves can be 15-20cm long and less than a centimeter wide. The leaves are alternate, sub-opposite in some cases, and arranged around the entire axis of the stem at the ends of the branches. The showy yellow flowers are funnel-shaped, approximately 6-10cm long by 3-5cm in diameter. Fruits are basically globose, but keeled which gives them a somewhat triangular shape depending on the angle. They are green to yellow, about 4-5cm in diameter, and hang in small clusters from individual stalks approximately 4-8cm long.

Uses: This plant is typically grown as an ornamental shrub, although it is poisonous due to the toxic latex. An extract of the leaves is used to treat toothaches and rheumatism, while material from the branches is used for fever and as a purgative (VDF). Yellow oleander has also been used to induce abortions and as an anesthetic, heart tonic, and to kill fish and insects (DAW).

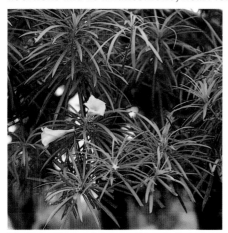

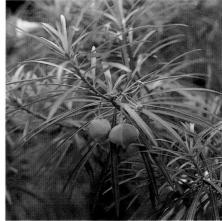

Fig. 217   Flowers, leaves, and developing fruits of yellow oleander (*Thevetia peruviana*).

Fig. 218   The pendulous fruits of yellow oleander.

Clove Vine
Clavo Huasca

Latin Name: ***Tynnanthus panurensis*** **(Bur.) Sandw.**
Bignoniaceae: Trumpet Vine or Catalpa Family

Description: This plant is a climbing vine that can grow to the size of a thick liana. It is named clove vine in both English and Spanish (*clavo* = clove, *huasca* = vine) due to the strong odor of cloves that is emitted from the stem, leaves, and sap. It has the typical opposite compound leaves found in the trumpet vine family, but they may have either two or three leaflets on the same plant. Leaflets are oval-shaped terminating in a definite drip-tip. Their margins are entire and may be slightly wavy. When two leaflets are present, they are equal in size; when trifoliate, the central or terminal leaflet is slightly larger. Leaflets generally range from 7-12cm long by 3-5cm wide. The petiole of the leaf is markedly longer than the petiolules of the lateral leaflets. The flowers are small and white and occur in clusters. The fruits are elongated flattened capsules, with the edges slightly raised.

Uses: Clove vine has three large cylindrical 'veins' that are extracted from the stem, chopped up, and mixed with *aguardiente* (sugar cane rum). This is taken to warm up a person, as well as used as a preventative (AMP). It is also used to impart energy and restore virility (AMP). Clove vine can also be prepared as a fragrant tea and used to treat rheumatism (AMP). The sap of this plant is used to treat fever (DAT). It has also been used for toothaches (JAD), although the clove oil used as a dental anesthetic and in mouthwashes in the developed world comes from a different plant family (Myrtaceae).

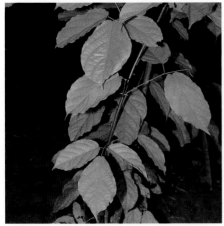

Fig. 219   Trifoliate leafves of the clove vine.

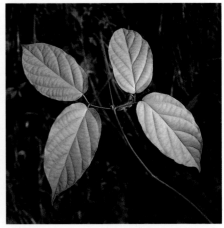

Fig. 220   A symmetrical pair of opposite leaves of clove vine, each with two leaflets.

Cat's Claw
Uña de Gato

Latin Name: *Uncaria* spp.
Rubiaceae: Madder or Coffee Family

Description: The cat's claw vine is a woody liana typically found in old
second growth forests. There are two species found in Central and South
America: *Uncaria guianensis* and *Uncaria tomentosa*. Older plants may
reach a girth of 20-30cm. They have simple, opposite, oval leaves with entire
margins that terminate in a point or short drip-tip. The leaves are usually 12-
16cm long by 5-7cm wide with a short (1cm or less) petiole. The leaves have
a few large secondary veins that alternate along the midvein, emerging in
diagonal fashion and curving up towards the tip as they approach the margin.
The most distinguishing feature is the paired, recurved spines for which the
plant is named. Both species are called cat's claw (*uña* = claw, *gato* = cat).
These 'claws' may be from 1-3cm long and occur at the nodes beneath the
leaves. They are a type of modified tendril adapted for support. The stems
of the newer growth are usually square. Round, dense flower heads 2-3cm in
diameter are typically produced in pairs at the nodes, one from each leaf axil,
on a 2-5cm long stalk. They may also form at the ends of branches. In *U.
tomentosa*, the blossoms are yellow-gold in color and give off a sweet odor
(TBC). The fruits of *U. tomentosa* are elliptical capsules clustered in round,
spiny-looking aggregations approximately 1-2cm in diameter (TBC). They
form a basket-like structure at maturity (TBC).

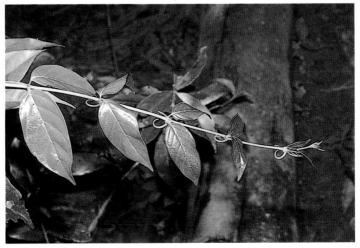

Fig. 221   A branch of the cat's claw vine (*Uncaria* sp.).

Uses: Cat's claw vines are well known throughout the tropics. The stem, bark, and leaves are traditionally used as a weak tea which has a slightly bitter taste and is taken regularly to prevent illness (AMP). The plant is also used to treat cancer, rheumatism, and internal wounds (AMP). A bark decoction of cat's claw has been used not only as an antiinflammatory agent and contraceptive, but also to treat stomach ulcers (VDF). In some areas it is believed to have curative powers over cancer infecting a woman's urinary tract (AED). Usage of cat's claw may also have rejuvenating potential (NIC). Advertisements in Peru now tout cat's claw extract as not only aiding with the previous maladies, but also in helping with arthritis, prostate and kidney problems, chronic tumors, ulcers, the elimination of acid urine, the bolstering of the immune system, and the prevention of AIDS. Most of these have yet to be proven, although there is a current worldwide market and cat's claw is exported in large quantities from Peru. It can be found in the Iquitos marketplace in either liquid form, or as a solid in small stacks of what resembles miniature cord wood. Commercial cat's claw tea bags are now marketed also.

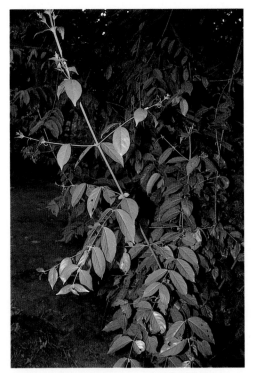

Fig. 222   Cat's claw grows as a woody liana or climbing vine (*Uncaria* sp.).

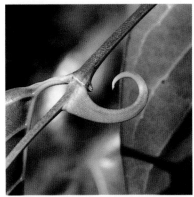

Fig. 223   Close-up of the spine or tendril of the cat's claw vine (*Uncaria* sp.)

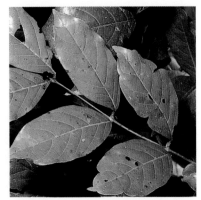

Fig. 224   The paired opposite leaves of the cat's claw vine (*Uncaria* sp.).

Jute
Yute

Latin Name: *Urena lobata* L.
Malvaceae: Mallow Family

Description: Jute is a weedy herb found throughout tropical and subtropical
regions in lowland habitats. It grows two to three meters high with very
straight, slender stems. It has simple alternate leaves that can vary greatly in
morphology and are borne on 3-5cm long petioles. Some are narrow and
strap-like, while others have three distinct deep lobes. Mature leaves are
approximately 12-20cm long by 2-4cm wide (unlobed) or 5-7cm wide (lobed).
The reticulate, indented venation gives the upper surface of the leaves a
wrinkled appearance, and the margins are slightly toothed.   The leaves bear a
longitudinal gland near the base of the midvein with a central slit in it (AHG).
The flowers are 3-4cm in diameter, borne in leaf axils, and consist of five
rounded pink petals and a maroon or purple center. The fruits are rounded
and sunken, with short spines, and about a half a centimeter in diameter
(AHG).

Uses: Jute is cultivated and harvested for its fiber, but should not be confused with the jute species (*Corchorus capsularis*) of worldwide commercial
importance. The latter belongs to a different plant family (Tiliaceae) and is
grown primarily in India and Bangladesh. *Urena lobata* has been cultivated
under plantation conditions in Brazil and Peru. The stems are harvested,
soaked in water, then stripped of their long fibers. These fibers are then hung
in the sun to dry. The result is a material similar to hemp.

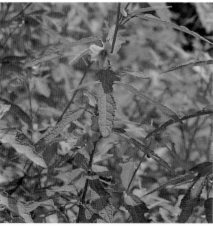

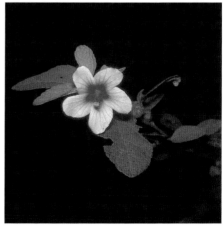

Fig. 225   Jute leaves and flowers (*Urena lobata*).   Fig. 226   Jute leaves and flower (*Urena lobata*).

Vanilla
Vainilla

Latin Name: *Vanilla planifolia* **Jacks. ex Andrews**
Orchidaceae: Orchid Family

Description: The vanilla orchid is a fleshy-stemmed, perennial, climbing vine. Wild-growing plants may get up to 20-30m long, using aerial roots to grow high up into the canopy. It is native to the lowland rainforests of Central America, northern South America, and the Caribbean. The leaves are alternate, thick and smooth, elongate with a slender oval shape, and with entire margins. Leaves usually range from 20-25cm long by 4-6cm wide and are constricted at the base. The flowers are large (7-10cm), yellow-green in color, and occur in groups of twenty or more. They last only a single day. In the wild, vanilla is only pollinated by a specific bee, and by several ant and hummingbird species. The fruit is a cylindrical capsule, 15-25cm in length, green, and resembles a string bean. These 'beans' mature in about nine months.

Uses: Vanilla was originally used as a flavoring by the Amerindians who cultivated it since before the Spanish explorers. It continues to be used as a flavoring in chocolate, desserts, ice cream, confections, as well as a scent in perfumes, tobaccos, and even as a stomach sedative. Pure vanilla extract is second only to saffron in cost due to the labor-intensive techniques necessary to cultivate and cure it. Cultivated vanilla must be trained on a trellis and hand-pollinated. The mature beans, once harvested, go through a process of curing, fermentation, and extraction that lasts for months. The major world producers of vanilla today are the Malagasy Republic and Indonesia.

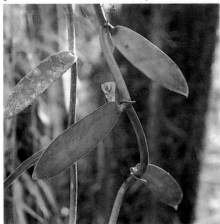

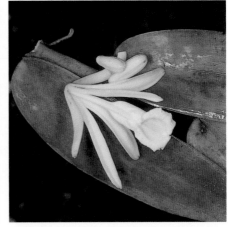

Fig. 227   Leaves and stem of the vanilla orchid (*Vanilla* sp.).

Fig. 228   Vanilla orchid in bloom (*Vanilla* sp.). (Photo by Mark Whitten)

Victoria Water Lily
Victoria Regia

Latin Name: *Victoria amazonica* (Poepp.) Sowerby
Nymphaeaceae: Water Lily Family

Description: This species along with *V. cruziana* make up the genus *Victoria*, which are giant water lilies. They are distributed throughout the tropical areas of South America. *V. amazonica* was formerly known as *V. regia* (the Queen Victoria lily), and may be found listed under that name in some references. This plant has a large round floating leaf, sometimes greater than a meter in diameter. The edge of the leaf is turned up for 5-10cm, perpendicular to the plane of the water. The top surface of the leaf is green, while the bottom is a dark purple. Main veins radiate out from the center of the leaf to the edge and are connected to one another by short crossveins. The sections delineated by veins are raised, more prominently so in younger, smaller leaves. The bottom surface is covered with large (2-4cm) spines, and the veins bulge out prominently. The large (20-30cm) white flowers open after dark and attract beetles that serve as pollinators, which are trapped when the flower closes before daylight. The color changes to purple during the day and the flower reopens at darkness releasing the beetles trapped within.

Uses: The root, stem, and seed of this plant are edible (RAR), the latter being high in starch (SAR). Aside from its ornamental appeal, material from *V. amazonica* is sometimes used as an additive when treating rheumatism, inflammation, and hemorrhoids (RVM). Another Spanish name for this plant is '*sábana del lagarto*' (*sábana* = sheet, *lagarto* = alligator) (AED).

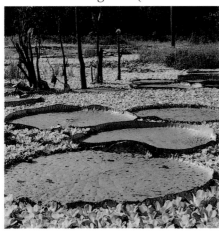

Fig. 229   Leaf of the Victoria water lily.

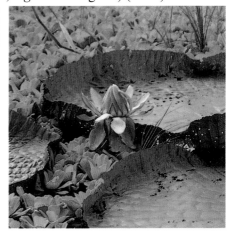

Fig. 230   Blossom of the Victoria water lily.

Virola
Cumala Blanca

Latin Name: *Virola* spp.
Myristicaceae: Nutmeg Family

Description: Most members of this family are trees, although some are
shrubs. The majority of species have a red latex. The leaves are alternate,
petiolate, oblong, margins entire, apex pointed, and with distinctive venation.
On younger trees, the branches are often characteristically whorled. The
fruits are fleshy and contain a large seed (= drupe). The seed is covered, at
least in part, by a fleshy thickening of the seed coat (= aril). (See photo of
opened virola fruit on page 11).

Uses: The inner bark of several species of this genus (*V. calophylla, V.
elongata*, and *V. surinamensis*) is grated into a powder and taken orally or
nasally for its powerful hallucinogenic effect. Preparations of *V. calophylla*
are also widely used by indigenous peoples to treat scabies and fungal problems (SAR). The latex of *V. elongata* is used for the latter as well (SAR).
A tea made from the leaves, latex, and bark of *V. surinamensis* is mixed with
Physalis angulata and used to treat stomachaches and inflammation (SAR).
The wood from a number of species of *Virola* is used for lumber (AED).
For additional information regarding the chemistry, preparation, and
hallucinogenic use of virola, see page 11.

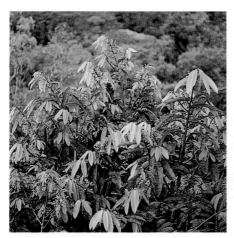 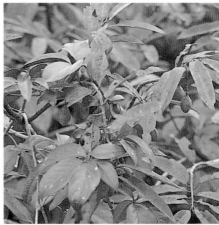

Fig. 231 *Virola* sp. in flower (Peru).
(Photo by Mark Plotkin)

Fig. 232 *Virola* sp. showing opened and
unopened fruits.   (Photo by Paul Donahue)

Vismia
Pichirina

Latin Name: *Vismia angusta* Miq.
Clusiaceae: Clusia Family

Description: This is a small tree of 5-10m height, usually found in second growth areas. The large simple opposite leaves are a distinctive, narrow, pointed, lance shape, and taper gradually from the base to apex. They resemble giant spear points. The older leaves may range from 35-50cm in length by 12-15cm width. The margins are entire and the petiole is short (2-3cm). The midvein is red to light brown in color, and the secondary veins are arranged alternate to subopposite from it. When a pair of new leaves emerges from the end of a branch, they are tightly appressed so that only their lower surfaces are showing. Such leaves are approximately 6-8cm long. They are a noticeably contrasting rich brown coppery color, as often is the new stem growth, due to a dense covering of small reddish-brown hairs. Similar coloration is seen in *Chrysophyllum cainito* (page 37). The overall appearance of the foliage caused by the large, paired lanceolate leaves with their copper-colored new growth makes this tree easy to identify, even when young. It produces an orange latex responsible for the name *sangre-gallina* (hen's blood).

Uses: The orange latex of this tree is used throughout the Amazon Basin by tribes for the treatment of sores and wounds (SAR). At least one group also uses it for lip herpes and skin fungus (SAR). The AED supports this, stating that the sap is used to treat ringworm (which is of fungal origin). The wood of this tree is also used for construction materials (AED).

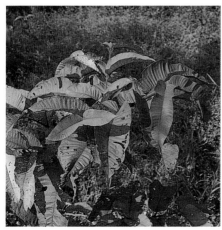

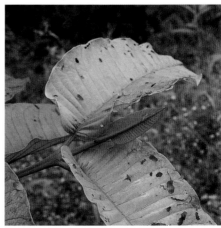

Fig. 233   Foliage of a young *Vismia angusta* tree.

Fig. 234   *Vismia angusta* showing copper-colored new leaves and branch.

Flag Tree
Bandera Caspi

Latin Name: *Warscewiczia coccinea* (Vahl) Klotzch
Rubiaceae: Madder or Coffee Family

Description: Flag tree is considered a subcanopy tree species, reaching a height of 12-15m. The long shiny leaves are opposite, simple, and entire. They are oval to elliptic in shape, and pointed at the apex. They range from 15-40cm long by 6-18cm wide with a short (2-3cm) petiole. There are many parallel secondary veins, depressed, giving the leaf surface a pleated appearance. The inflorescence consists of paired, regularly-spaced, dense clusters of small yellow flowers on a long (up to 80cm) straight rachis from the end of the branch. Projecting laterally from this rachis beyond the yellow, centrally-located blossoms are large, bright red, leaf-like bracts. These are oval with several longitudinal veins, about 12cm long by 4cm wide, and with a long (4-6cm) narrow petiole-like base. The yellow flowers and red bracts resemble a linear poinsettia. The fruits are roundish capsules about .5cm long. (TBC). The plants are characteristic of disturbed sites, and found near streams.

Uses: The dried, powdered root of flag tree is used in traditional medicine as a treatment for fungal dermatitis (SAR). The root is boiled and rubbed on the back to help alleviate back pain (SAR). Pieces of the root are worn by some Indians as a source of perfume and aphrodisiac (JAD), while a drink from the cooked root is taken for persistent nosebleed (FOR). This tree is also grown solely for its ornamental value due to its colorful and showy inflorescences.

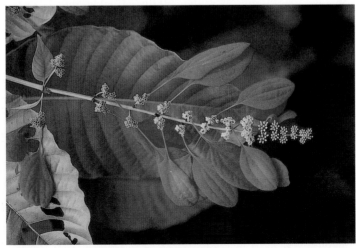

Fig. 235   Terminal inflorescence of the flag tree.

Ginger
Jengibre

Latin Name: ***Zingiber officinale*** **Roscoe**
Zingiberaceae: Ginger Family

Description: Ginger is not native to the New World, but is now grown throughout the tropics. It is an aromatic herb that reaches a height of slightly more than one meter. The alternately arranged leaves occur in two rows on opposite sides of a fleshy stem. The leaves are simple, long and narrow, coming to a slender point at the apex. The edges are entire and their bases sheath the stem. The leaves narrow at the base, but lack a petiole. They range in size from about 12-25cm long by 2-3cm wide. Only the lighter colored midvein is easily visible. The inflorescence is spike-like and usually is produced on a stalk coming from the root, but in some cases can be found originating from the stem. It is found at a level shorter than the other stems of the plant. The end of the flower stalk is swollen and green, about 5-7cm long by 2-3cm wide and produces yellow and purple flowers. The underground portion of the plant is a swollen rhizome that is aromatic.

Uses: This plant is the souce of commercial ginger which is used as a spice and flavoring agent. It is derived from the dried or fresh rhizome. The crushed rhizomes in *aguardiente* are taken for rheumatism and arthritis, and to increase virility (AED). The rhizomes are also used for diarrhea and stomachaches (AED), headaches (GMJ), and bronchitis (RVM). Extracts have shown antiinflammatory activity comparable to aspirin (TRA). Indian women use a tea for sore throat, colic, and menstrual cramps (AED).

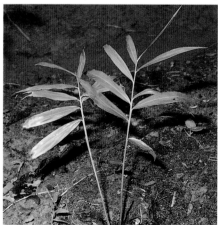

Fig. 236 Growth habit of ginger (*Zingiber officinale*).

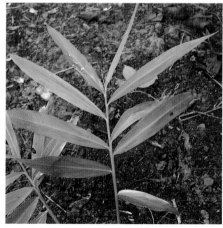

Fig. 237 Leaves of ginger (*Zingiber officinale*).

Bibliography

The following three titles were consulted extensively while researching this book.

Amazonian Ethnobotanical Dictionary
James A. Duke and Rodolfo Vasquez
CRC Press   (Boca Raton, Florida)
1994   ISBN 0-8493-3664-3

The Healing Forest
Richard E. Schultes and Robert F. Raffauf
Dioscorides Press   (Portland, Oregon)
1990   ISBN 0-931146-14-3

Woody Plants Of Northwest South America
Alwyn H. Gentry
University of Chicago Press   (Chicago, Illinois)
1993   ISBN 0-226-28944-3

The next six titles were also extremely useful references.

Flora Of Barro Colorado Island
Thomas B. Croat
Stanford University Press   (Stanford, California)
1978   ISBN 0-8047-0950-5

Cultivo De Frutales Nativos Amazónicos
Tratado De Cooperación Amazonica (TCA)
IIAP, UNDP, FAO   (Lima, Peru)
1997   SPT-TCA / No. 51

Field Guide To The Palms Of The Americas
Andrew Henderson, Gloria Galeano, and Rodrigo Bernal
Princeton University Press   (Princeton, New Jersey)
1995   ISBN 0-691-01600-3

Rainforest Remedies
Rosita Arvigo and Michael Balick
Lotus Press   (Twin Lakes, Wisconsin)
1993   ISBN 0-914955-13-6

Tropical Forests And Their Crops
Nigel J.H. Smith, J.T. Williams, Donald L. Plucknett, and Jennifer P. Talbot
Cornell University Press   (Ithaca, New York)
1992   ISBN 0-8014-8058-2

Economic Botany: Plants In Our World
Beryl B. Simpson and Molly C. Ogorzaly
McGraw-Hill   (New York, New York)
1995   ISBN 0-07-057569-X

The remaining titles are listed alphabetically by the author's name and deal with medicinal/hallucinogenic plants, and tropical fruits and forests.

Rainforest Remedies
Rosita Arvigo and Michael Balick
Lotus Press   (Twin Lakes, Wisconsin)
1993   ISBN 0-914955-13-6

Notes On Some Medicinal And Poisonous Plants Of Amazonian Peru
Flore F. Ayala
Advances in Economic Botany 1: 1-8. 1984

Jungles
Edward Ayensu (Editor)
Crown Publishers   (New York, New York)
1980   ISBN 0-517-54136X

Useful Plants of Amazonia
Michael J. Balick   (Chapter 19)
Ghillean T. Prance and Thomas E. Lovejoy (Editors)
Pergamon Press
1985

Folk Medicine of Alter do Chão, Pará, Brazil
L.C. Branch and I.M.F. da Silva
Acta Amazonica 13(5/6): 737-797. 1983

Medicinal Resources Of The Tropical Forest
Michael J. Balick, Elaine Elisabetsky, and Sarah A. Laird (Editors)
Columbia University Press   (New York, New York)
1996   ISBN 0-231-10171-6

Healing Herbs
Michael Castleman
Bantam Books   (New York, New York)
1995   ISBN 0-553-56988-0

Frutas Comestíveis da Amazônia (in Portuguese)
Paulo B. Cavalcante
Museu Paraense Emilio Goeldi   (Belém, Brazil)
1988   ISBN 85-7098-009-4

List Of Plants Used By The Indigenous Chami Of Riseralda (in Spanish)
A.E. Cayon and G.S. Arisitizabal
Cespedesia 9(33-4): 5-15. 1980

Flora Of Barro Colorado Island
Thomas B. Croat
Stanford University Press   (Stanford, California)
1978   ISBN 0-8047-0950-5

Cultivo De Frutales Nativos Amazónicos (in Spanish)
Tratado De Cooperación Amazonica (TCA)
IIAP, UNDP, FAO   (Lima, Peru)
1997   SPT-TCA / No. 51

One River
Wade Davis
Simon and Schuster   (New York, New York)
1996   ISBN 0-684-83496-0

Swidden-Fallow Agroforestry In The Peruvian Amazon
W.M. Denevan and Padoch, C.
Advances In Economic Botany 5: 8-46. 1988

Medicinal Plants Of The World (computer index)
J.A. Duke and K.K. Wain

Medicinal And Magical Plants In The Northern Peruvian Andes
V. de Feo
Fitoterapia 63: 417-440. 1992

Ethnobotany Of The Cuna & Waunana Indigenous Communities, Choco
P.L.E. Forero
Cespedesia 9(33): 115-302. 1980

138

Chilies To Chocolate
Nelson Foster and Linda S. Cordell (Editors)
University of Arizona Press   (Tucson, Arizona)
1992   ISBN 0-8165-1324-4

Woody Plants Of Northwest South America
Alwyn H. Gentry
University of Chicago Press   (Chicago, Illinois)
1993   ISBN 0-226-28944-3

Frutas En Colombia (in Spanish)
Eduardo Sarmiento Gomez
Ediciones Cultural Colombiana   (Bogota, Colombia)
1986   ISBN 958-9013-30-9

Pharmacopées Taditionnels En Guyane: Créoles, Palikur, Wayãpi
P. Grenand, C. Moretti, and H. Jacquemin   (in French)
Editorial 1-ORSTOM, Coll. Mem. No. 108, Paris. 1987

*Plantas De Uso Medicinal, Mágico Y Psicotrópico
       Del Estado Amazonas, Venezuela* (in Spanish)
Francisco Guanchez
PNUD-SADA. AMAZONAS
Fundación Polar (Caracas, Venezuela)
In Press (1998)

Field Guide To The Palms Of The Americas
Andrew Henderson, Gloria Galeano, and Rodrigo Bernal
Princeton University Press   (Princeton, New Jersey)
1995   ISBN 0-691-01600-3

The Fruit Expert
D.G. Hessayon
Transworld Publishers   (London, England)
1995   ISBN 0-903505-31-2

Wizard Of The Upper Amazon
F. Bruce Lamb
North Atlantic Books   (Berkeley, California)
1974   ISBN 0-938190-80-6

Plants For People
Anna Lewington
Oxford University Press   (New York, New York)
1990   ISBN 0-19-520840-4

Witch-Doctor's Apprentice
Nicole Maxwell
Citadell Press   (New York, New York)
1990   ISBN 0-8065-1174-5

Tropical Rainforest
Arnold Newman
Facts On File   (New York, New York)
1990   ISBN 0-8160-1944-4

Plantas Útiles De Colombia (in Spanish)
E. Perez-Arbelaez
Librería Colombiana   (Bogotá, Colombia)
1956

Tales Of A Shaman's Apprentice
Mark J. Plotkin
Penguin Books   (New York, New York)
1993   ISBN 0-14-012991-X

The Shaman's Apprentice (Children's Version)
Lynne Cherry and Mark J. Plotkin
Harcourt Brace & Co.   (San Diego, California)
1998   ISBN 0-15-201281-8

Marvels Of Our Medicinal Flora (in Spanish)
L.J. Poveda
Biocenosis Volumes 1 & 2. 1985-86

Arvores De Manaus (in Portuguese)
G. T. Prance and M. F. Silva
Instituto Nacional de Pesquisas da Amazonia (Manaus, Brazil)
1975

Catálogo De Plantas Útiles De La Amazonia Peruana
Richard A. Rutter
1990   Summer Institute of Linguistics

The Healing Forest
Richard E. Schultes and Robert F. Raffauf
Dioscorides Press   (Portland, Oregon)
1990   ISBN 0-931146-14-3

Vine Of The Soul
Richard E. Schultes and Robert F. Raffauf
Synergetic Press   (Synerg, Arizona)
1992   ISBN 0-907791-24-7

Towards A Caribbean Pharmacopoeia
L. Robineau (Ed.)
Based on Tramil Workshop: Scientific Research and Popular Use of Medicinal Plants in the Caribbean #4, 1989, Tela, Honduras.
Enda Caribbe, Santo Domingo. 474 pp.

The Great Exotic Fruit Book
Norman Van Aken with John Harrisson
Ten Speed Press   (Berkeley, California)
1995   ISBN 0-89815-688-2

A Field Guide To Medicinal And Useful Plants Of The Upper Amazon
James L. Castner, Stephen L. Timme and James A. Duke
Feline Press   (Gainesville, Florida)
1998   ISBN 0-9625150-7-8

The following is a free search service that will locate hard to find or out of print books for you with no obligation to buy.

Out-Of-State Book Service
Box 3253
San Clemente, CA 92674-3253
Phone: 714-492-2976

Specialty Organizations with Related Books or Products For Sale

American Botanical Council
P.O. Box 201660
Austin, TX   78720-1660
Phone: (512)-331-8868
e-mail: abc@herbalgram.org
Web Site: http://www.herbalgram.org

South American Explorers Club
126 Indian Creek Road
Ithaca, N.Y. 14850
Phone: (607)-277-0488
e-mail: explorer@samexplo.org
Web Site: http://www.samexplo.org

Patricia Ledlie Bookseller, Inc.
One Bean Road
P.O. Box 90
Buckfield, ME 04220
Phone: (800)-791-1028
e-mail: ledlie@ledlie.com
Web Site: http://www.ledlie.com

Balogh Scientific Books
1911 N. Duncan Road
Champaign, IL 61821
Phone: (217)-355-9331
e-mail: balogh@balogh.com
Web Site: http://www.balogh.com

The Latin American Book Store
204 North Geneva Street
Ithaca, N.Y. 14850
Phone: (607)-273-2418
e-mail: libros@latinamericanbooks.com
Web Site: http://www.latinamericanbooks.com

Flo Silver Books
8442 Oakwood Court North
Indianapolis, IN 46260
Phone: (317)-255-5118
e-mail: Flosilver@aol.com

Native Habitat Ethnobotanicals
P.O. Box 644023
Vero Beach, FL 32964-4023
e-mail: NHE@juno.com
Web Site: http://www.nativehabitat.com

Summer Institute of Linguistics
International Academic Bookstore
7500 West Camp Wisdom Road
Dallas, TX 75236-5626
Phone: (214)-709-2404
e-mail: academic.books@sil.org

Ediciones Abya-Yala
Avenida 12 de Octubre 1430 y Wilson
Casilla 17-12-719
Quito, Ecuador
Phone: 506-267 or 562-633 or 506-247
e-mail: Abyayala@abyayala.org.ec

Feline Press
P.O. Box 7219
Gainesville, FL 32605 USA
e-mail: jlcastner@aol.com

Herbal Vineyard, Inc.
8210 Murphy Road
Fulton, MD 20759
e-mail: jimduke@cpcug.org
URL for Father Nature's Farmacy
http://www.ars-grin.gov/~ngrlsb/

Plant Species By Latin Name

Page	Latin Name	English Name	Spanish Name
13	*Abuta grandifolia*	abuta	motelo sanango
14	*Anacardium occidentale*	cashew	cashu, marañón
16	*Ananas comosus*	pineapple	piña
17	*Arrabidaea chica*	dye plant	puca panga
18	*Artocarpus altilis*	breadfruit	pan del árbol
19	*Asclepias curassavica*	tropical milkweed	flor de muerto
20	*Averrhoa carambola*	star fruit	carambola
21	*Banisteriopsis caapi*	soul vine	ayahuasca, yagé
22	*Bauhinia guianensis*	monkey ladder	escalera de mono
23	*Bellucia* sp.	nispero	níspero
24	*Bertholletia excelsa*	Brazil nut	castaña
25	*Bidens alba*	Spanish needles	amor seco
26	*Bixa orellana*	annatto	achiote
28	*Brugmansia suaveolens*	angel's trumpet	toé
29	*Brunfelsia grandiflora*	fever tree	chiric sanango
30	*Caesalpinia pulcherrima*	pride of Barbados	angel sisa
31	*Calycophyllum* spp.	firewood tree	capirona
31	*Capirona* spp.	firewood tree	capirona
32	*Carica papaya*	papaya	papaya
33	*Carludovica palmata*	Panama hat 'palm'	bombonaje
34	*Ceiba pentandra*	kapok	lupuna, ceiba
35	*Chenopodium*	wormseed	paico *ambrosioides*
36	*Chondrodendron*	curare	curaré *tomentosum*
37	*Chrysophyllum cainito*	caimito	caimito
38	*Cissus sicyoides*	toad vine	sapo huasca
39	*Clusia rosea*	clusia	renaquilla
40	*Coffea* spp.	coffee	café
42	*Costus lasius*	pineapple ginger	cañagre
43	*Costus scaber*	candlestick ginger	cañagre
44	*Couma macrocarpa*	milk tree	leche caspi
45	*Crescentia cujete*	calabash	huingo
46	*Croton lechleri*	dragon's blood	sangre del grado
47	*Curcuma longa*	turmeric	guisador
48	*Cymbopogon citratus*	lemon grass	hierba luisa
49	*Dracontium loretense*	fer-de-lance plant	jergón sacha
50	*Eryngium foetidum*	wild coriander	sacha culantro
51	*Erythrina fusca*	swamp immortelle	amasisa
52	*Erythroxylon coca*	coca, cocaine plant	coca
53	*Eucharis castelnaeana*	Amazon lily	delia
54	*Ficus insipida*	medicinal fig	ojé

Plant Species By Latin Name

Page	Latin Name	English Name	Spanish Name
55	*Genipa americana*	genipap	huito
56	*Gossypium* spp.	cotton	algodón
57	*Grias neuberthii*	wild mango	sacha mango
58	*Heliotropium indicum*	heliotrope	alacransillo
59	*Helosis guyannensis*	blood 'mushroom'	aguajillo
60	*Hevea brasiliensis*	rubber	shiringa
62	*Himatanthus sucuuba*	himatanthus	bellaco caspi
63	*Inga edulis*	ice cream bean	guaba, shimbillo
64	*Ipomoea batatas*	sweet potato	camote
65	*Ipomoea quamoclit*	cypress vine	enredadera
66	*Iriartea deltoidea*	stilt palm	huacrapona
67	*Jatropha curcas*	physic nut	piñón blanco
68	*Jatropha gossypifolia*	black physic nut	piñón negro
69	*Kalanchoe pinnata*	air plant	hoja de aire
70	*Lantana camara*	lantana	aya albaca
71	*Lepianthes peltata*	Santa Maria	Santa María
72	*Lepidocaryum tenue*	thatch palm	irapay
73	*Lippia alba*	lippia	pampa orégano
74	*Maclura tinctoria*	toothache tree	insira amarilla
75	*Mangifera indica*	mango	mango
76	*Manihot esculenta*	cassava, manioc	yuca
78	*Manilkara zapota*	chewing gum tree	sapodilla
79	*Mansoa alliacea*	wild garlic	ajo sacha
80	*Maquira coriacea*	capinuri	capinurí
81	*Mauritia flexuosa*	moriche palm	aguaje
82	*Melia azedarach*	China berry	paraíso
83	*Mimosa pudica*	sensitive plant	chami
84	*Mucuna rostrata*	mucuna	vaca ñahui
85	*Musa* spp.	banana, plantain	banano, plátano
86	*Myrciaria cauliflora*	jaboticaba	jaboticaba
87	*Myrciaria dubia*	camu camu	camu camu
88	*Ochroma pyrimidale*	balsa	balsa
89	*Ocimum micranthum*	wild basil	pichana albaca
90	*Oryza sativa*	rice	arroz
92	*Passiflora coccinea*	red passion vine	granadilla venenosa
93	*Passiflora edulis*	purple passion vine	maracuyá
94	*Passiflora quadrangularis*	giant granadilla	tumbo
95	*Paullinia cupana*	guarana	guaraná
96	*Persea americana*	avocado	palta, aguacate
97	*Petiveria alliacea*	garlic weed	mucura

Plant Species By Latin Name

Page	Latin Name	English Name	Spanish Name
98	*Phyllanthus niruri*	stonebreaker	chanca piedra
99	*Phytelephas aequatorialis*	ivory palm	yarina, tagua
100	*Phytolacca rivinoides*	pokeberry	jaboncillo
101	*Piper* sp.	shoestring pepper	cordoncillo
102	*Pistia stratiotes*	water lettuce	huama
103	*Plumeria alba*	frangipani	suche rosado
104	*Portulaca oleracea*	purslane	verdolaga
105	*Potalia amara*	snakebite plant	curarina
106	*Psidium guajava*	guava	guayabo
107	*Psychotria* spp.	psychotria	yagé
108	*Renealmia alpinia*	dwarf ginger	mishquipanga enano
109	*Ricinus communis*	castor bean	higuerilla
110	*Saccharum officinarum*	sugar cane	caña de azúcar
112	*Scoparia dulcis*	sweet broom	ñucñupichana
113	*Selaginella* spp.	spike moss	shapumba
114	*Senna reticulata*	wild senna	retama amarilla
115	*Simarouba amara*	simarouba	marupá
116	*Siparuna guianensis*	siparuna	picho huayo
117	*Socratea exorrhiza*	stilt palm	pona
118	*Solanum mammosum*	breast berry	cocona venenosa
119	*Solanum obliquum*	tree tomato	gallinazo panga
120	*Solanum sessiliflorum*	cocona	cocona
121	*Strychnos guianensis*	strychnine	comida del venado
122	*Theobroma cacao*	cocoa, chocolate tree	cacao
124	*Thevetia peruviana*	yellow oleander	camalonga
125	*Tynnanthus panurensis*	clove vine	clavo huasca
126	*Uncaria* spp.	cat's claw vine	uña de gato
128	*Urena lobata*	jute	yute
129	*Vanilla planifolia*	vanilla	vainilla
130	*Victoria amazonica*	Victoria water lily	victoria regia
131	*Virola* spp.	virola	cumala blanca
132	*Vismia angusta*	vismia	pichirina
133	*Warscewiczia coccinea*	flag tree	bandera caspi
134	*Zingiber officinale*	ginger	jengibre

Plant Species By English Name

Page	English Name	Latin Name	Spanish Name
13	abuta	*Abuta grandifolia*	motelo sanango
69	air plant	*Kalanchoe pinnata*	hoja de aire
53	Amazon lily	*Eucharis castelnaeana*	delia
28	angel's trumpet	*Brugmansia suaveolens*	toé
26	annatto	*Bixa orellana*	achiote
96	avocado	*Persea americana*	aguacate, palta
88	balsa	*Ochroma pyrimidale*	balsa
85	banana	*Musa* sp.	banano
68	black physic nut	*Jatropha gossypifolia*	piñón negro
59	blood 'mushroom'	*Helosis guyannensis*	aguajillo
24	Brazil nut tree	*Bertholletia excelsa*	castaña
18	breadfruit	*Artocarpus altilis*	pan del árbol
118	breast berry	*Solanum mammosum*	cocona venenosa
37	caimito	*Chrysophyllum cainito*	caimito
45	calabash	*Crescentia cujete*	huingo
87	camu camu	*Myrciaria dubia*	camu camu
43	candlestick ginger	*Costus scaber*	cañagre
80	capinuri	*Maquira coriacea*	capinurí
14	cashew	*Anacardium occidentale*	cashu, marañon
76	cassava	*Manihot esculenta*	yuca
109	castor bean	*Ricinus communis*	higuerilla
126	cat's claw vine	*Uncaria* spp.	uña de gato
78	chewing gum tree	*Manilkara zapota*	sapodilla
82	China berry	*Melia azedarach*	paraíso
122	chocolate tree	*Theobroma cacao*	cacao
125	clove vine	*Tynnanthus panurensis*	clavo huasca
52	cocaine bush	*Erythroxylon coca*	coca
122	cocoa	*Theobroma cacao*	cacao
120	cocona	*Solanum sessiliflorum*	cocona
40	coffee	*Coffea* spp.	café
56	cotton	*Gossypium* spp.	algodón
36	curare	*Chondrodendron*	curaré
			tomentosum
65	cypress vine	*Ipomoea quamoclit*	enredadera
46	dragon's blood	*Croton lechleri*	sangre del grado
108	dwarf ginger	*Renealmia alpinia*	mishquipanga enano
17	dye plant	*Arribadaea chica*	puca panga
49	fer-de-lance plant	*Dracontium loretense*	jergón sacha
29	fever tree	*Brunfelsia grandiflora*	chiric sanango
31	firewood tree	*Calycophyllum* spp.	capirona
		Capirona spp.	capirona
133	flag tree	*Warsczewiczia coccinea*	bandera caspi

Plant Species By English Name

Pages	English Name	Latin Name	Spanish Name
103	frangipani	*Plumeria alba*	suche rosado
97	garlic weed	*Petiveria alliacea*	mucura
55	genipap	*Genipa americana*	huito
94	giant granadilla	*Passiflora quadrangularis*	tumbo
134	ginger	*Zingiber officinale*	jengibre
95	guarana	*Paullinia cupana*	guaraná
106	guava	*Psidium guajava*	guayabo
58	heliotrope	*Heliotropium indicum*	alacransillo
62	himatanthus	*Himatanthus sucuuba*	bellaco caspi
63	ice cream bean	*Inga edulis*	guaba, shimbillo
99	ivory palm	*Phytelephas aequatorialis*	yarina, tagua
86	jaboticaba	*Myrciaria cauliflora*	jaboticaba
128	jute	*Urena lobata*	yute
34	kapok	*Ceiba pentandra*	lupuna, ceiba
70	lantana	*Lantana camara*	aya albaca
48	lemon grass	*Cymbopogon citratus*	hierba luisa
73	lippia	*Lippia alba*	pampa orégano
75	mango	*Mangifera indica*	mango
76	manioc	*Manihot esculenta*	yuca
54	medicinal fig	*Ficus insipida*	ojé
44	milk tree	*Couma macrocarpa*	leche caspi
22	monkey ladder	*Bauhinia guianensis*	escalera de mono
81	moriche palm	*Mauritia flexuosa*	aguaje
84	mucuna	*Mucuna rostrata*	vaca ñahui
23	nispero	*Bellucia* spp.	níspero
33	Panama hat 'palm'	*Carludovica palmata*	bombonaje
32	papaya	*Carica papaya*	papaya
67	physic nut	*Jatropha curcas*	piñón blanco
16	pineapple	*Ananas comosus*	piña
42	pineapple ginger	*Costus lasius*	cañagre
85	plantain	*Musa* sp.	plátano
100	pokeberry	*Phytolacca rivinoides*	jaboncillo
30	pride of Barbados	*Caesalpinia pulcherrima*	angel sisa
107	psychotria	*Psychotria* spp.	yagé
93	purple passion vine	*Passiflora edulis*	maracuyá
104	purslane	*Portulaca oleracea*	verdolaga
92	red passion vine	*Passiflora coccinea*	granadilla venenosa

Plant Species By English Name

Pages	English Name	Latin Name	Spanish Name
90	rice	*Oryza sativa*	arroz
60	rubber	*Hevea brasiliensis*	shiringa
71	Santa Maria	*Lepianthes peltata*	Santa María
83	sensitive plant	*Mimosa pudica*	chami
101	shoestring pepper	*Piper* sp.	cordoncillo
115	simarouba	*Simarouba amara*	marupá
116	siparuna	*Siparuna guianensis*	picho huayo
105	snakebite plant	*Potalia amara*	curarina
21	soul vine	*Banisteriopsis caapi*	ayahuasca
25	Spanish needles	*Bidens alba*	amor seco
113	spike moss	*Selaginella* spp.	shapumba
39	star fruit	*Clusia rosea*	renaquilla
20	star fruit	*Averrhoa carambola*	carambola
117	stilt palm	*Socratea exorrhiza*	pona
66	stilt palm	*Iriartea deltoidea*	huacrapona
98	stonebreaker	*Phyllanthus niruri*	chanca piedra
121	strychnine plant	*Strychnos guianensis*	comida del venado
110	sugar cane	*Saccharum officinarum*	caña de azúcar
51	swamp immortelle	*Erythrina fusca*	amasisa
112	sweet broom	*Scoparia dulcis*	ñucñupichana
64	sweet potato	*Ipomoea batatas*	camote
72	thatch palm	*Lepidocaryum tenue*	irapay
38	toad vine	*Cissus sicyoides*	sapo huasca
74	toothache tree	*Maclura tinctoria*	insira amarilla
119	tree tomato	*Solanum obliquum*	gallinazo panga
19	tropical milkweed	*Asclepias curassavica*	flor de muerto
47	turmeric	*Curcuma longa*	guisador
129	vanilla	*Vanilla planifolia*	vainilla
130	Victoria water lily	*Victoria amazonica*	victoria regia
131	virola	*Virola* spp.	cumala blanca
132	vismia	*Vismia angusta*	pichirina
102	water lettuce	*Pistia stratiotes*	huama
89	wild basil	*Ocimum micranthum*	pichana albaca
50	wild coriander	*Eryngium foetidum*	sacha culantro
79	wild garlic	*Mansoa alliacea*	ajo sacha
57	wild mango	*Grias neuberthii*	sacha mango
114	wild senna	*Senna reticulata*	retama amarilla
35	wormseed	*Chenopodium ambrosioides*	paico
124	yellow oleander	*Thevetia peruviana*	camalonga

Plant Species By Spanish Name

Pages	Spanish Name	Latin Name	English Name
13	abuta	*Abuta grandifolia*	abuta
26	achiote	*Bixa orellana*	annatto
96	aguacate	*Persea americana*	avocado
81	aguaje	*Mauritia flexuosa*	moriche palm
59	aguajillo	*Helosis guyannensis*	'blood' mushroom
79	ajo sacha	*Mansoa alliacea*	wild garlic
58	alacransillo	*Heliotropium indicum*	heliotrope
56	algodón	*Gossypium* spp.	cotton
51	amasisa	*Erythrina fusca*	swamp immortelle
25	amor seco	*Bidens alba*	Spanish needles
30	angel sisa	*Caesalpinia pulcherrima*	pride of Barbados
90	arroz	*Oryza sativa*	rice
21	ayahuasca	*Banisteriopsis caapi*	soul vine
70	aya albaca	*Lantana camara*	lantana
88	balsa	*Ochroma pyrimidale*	balsa
85	banano	*Musa* sp.	banana
133	bandera caspi	*Warscewiczia coccinea*	flag tree
62	bellaco caspi	*Himatanthus sucuuba*	himatanthus
33	bombonaje	*Carludovica palmata*	Panama hat 'palm'
122	cacao	*Theobroma cacao*	cocoa, chocolate
40	café	*Coffea* spp.	coffee
37	caimito	*Chrysophyllum cainito*	caimito
124	camalonga	*Thevetia peruviana*	yellow oleander
64	camote	*Ipomoea batatas*	sweet potato
87	camu camu	*Myrciaria dubia*	camu camu
110	caña de azúcar	*Saccharum officinarum*	sugar cane
42	cañagre	*Costus lasius*	pineapple ginger
43	cañagre	*Costus scaber*	candlestick ginger
80	capinurí	*Maquira coriacea*	capinuri
31	capirona	*Calycophyllum* spp.	firewood tree
31	capirona	*Capirona* spp.	firewood tree
20	carambola	*Averrhoa carambola*	star fruit
14	cashu	*Anacardium occidentale*	cashew
76	cassava	*Manihot esculenta*	cassava
24	castaña	*Bertholletia excelsa*	Brazil nut
34	ceiba	*Ceiba pentandra*	kapok
125	clavo huasca	*Tynnanthus panurensis*	clove vine
52	coca	*Erythroxylon coca*	coca, cocaine bush
120	cocona	*Solanum sessiliflorum*	cocona
118	cocona venenosa	*Solanum mammosum*	breast berry
121	comida del venado	*Strychnos guianensis*	strychnine

Plant Species By Spanish Name

Pages	Spanish Name	Latin Name	English Name
101	cordoncillo	*Piper* sp.	shoestring pepper
131	cumala blanca	*Virola* spp.	virola
36	curaré	*Chondrodendron tomentosum*	curare
105	curarina	*Potalia amara*	snakebite plant
83	chami	*Mimosa pudica*	sensitive plant
98	chanca piedra	*Phyllanthus niruri*	stonebreaker
29	chiric sanango	*Brunfelsia grandiflora*	fever tree
53	delia	*Eucharis castelnaeana*	Amazon lily
65	enredadera	*Ipomoea quamoclit*	cypress vine
22	escalera de mono	*Bauhinia guianensis*	monkey ladder
19	flor de muerto	*Asclepias curassavica*	tropical milkweed
119	gallinazo panga	*Solanum obliquum*	tree tomato
92	granadilla venenosa	*Passiflora coccinea*	red passion vine
63	guaba	*Inga edulis*	ice cream bean
47	guisador	*Curcuma longa*	turmeric
95	guaraná	*Paullinia cupana*	guarana
106	guayabo	*Psidium guajava*	guava
48	hierba luisa	*Cymbopogon citratus*	lemon grass
109	higuerilla	*Ricinus communis*	castor bean
69	hoja de aire	*Kalanchoe pinnata*	air plant
66	huacrapona	*Iriartea deltoidea*	stilt palm
102	huama	*Pistia stratiotes*	water lettuce
45	huingo	*Crescentia cujete*	calabash
55	huito	*Genipa americana*	genipap
74	insira amarilla	*Maclura tinctoria*	toothache tree
72	irapay	*Lepidocaryum tenue*	thatch palm
100	jaboncillo	*Phytolacca rivinoides*	pokeberry
86	jaboticaba	*Myrciaria cauliflora*	jaboticaba
134	jengibre	*Zingiber officinale*	ginger
49	jergón sacha	*Dracontium loretense*	fer-de-lance plant
44	leche caspi	*Couma macrocarpa*	milk tree
34	lupuna	*Ceiba pentandra*	kapok
75	mango	*Mangifera indica*	mango
93	maracuyá	*Passiflora edulis*	purple passion vine
14	marañón	*Anacardium occidentale*	cashew
115	marupá	*Simarouba amara*	simarouba
108	mishquipanga enano	*Renealmia alpinia*	dwarf ginger
97	mucura	*Petiveria alliacea*	garlic weed
23	níspero	*Bellucia* spp.	nispero
112	ñucñupichana	*Scoparia dulcis*	sweet broom

Plant Species By Spanish Name

Pages	Spanish Name	Latin Name	English Name
54	ojé	*Ficus insipida*	medicinal fig
35	paico	*Chenopodium ambrosioides*	wormseed
96	palta	*Persea americana*	avocado
73	pampa orégano	*Lippia alba*	lippia
18	pan del árbol	*Artocarpus altilis*	breadfruit
32	papaya	*Carica papaya*	papaya
82	paraíso	*Melia azedarach*	China berry
89	pichana albaca	*Ocimum micranthum*	wild basil
132	pichirina	*Vismia angusta*	vismia
116	picho huayo	*Siparuna guianensis*	siparuna
16	piña	*Ananas comosus*	pineapple
67	piñón blanco	*Jatropha curcas*	physic nut
68	piñón negro	*Jatropha gossypifolia*	black physic nut
85	plátano	*Musa* sp.	plantain
117	pona	*Socratea exorrhiza*	stilt palm
17	puca panga	*Arrabidaea chica*	dye plant
39	renaquilla	*Clusia rosea*	star fruit
114	retama amarilla	*Senna reticulata*	wild senna
50	sacha culantro	*Eryngium foetidum*	wild coriander
57	sacha mango	*Grias neuberthii*	wild mango
46	sangre del grado	*Croton lechleri*	dragon's blood
71	Santa María	*Lepianthes peltata*	Santa Maria
78	sapodilla	*Manilkara zapota*	chewing gum tree
38	sapo huasca	*Cissus sicyoides*	toad vine
113	shapumba	*Selaginella exaltata*	spike moss
63	shimbillo	*Inga edulis*	ice cream bean
60	shiringa	*Hevea brasiliensis*	rubber
103	suche rosado	*Plumeria alba*	frangipani
99	tagua	*Phytelephas aequatorialis*	ivory palm
28	toé	*Brugmansia suaveolens*	angel's trumpet
94	tumbo	*Passiflora quadrangularis*	giant granadilla
126	uña de gato	*Uncaria* spp.	cat's claw vine
84	vaca ñahui	*Mucuna rostrata*	mucuna
129	vainilla	*Vanilla planifolia*	vanilla
104	verdolaga	*Portulaca oleracea*	purslane
130	victoria regia	*Victoria amazonica*	Victoria water lily
107	yagé	*Psychotria* sp.	psychotria
99	yarina	*Phytelephas aequatorialis*	ivory palm
76	yuca	*Manihot esculenta*	cassava, manioc
128	yute	*Urena lobata*	jute

James L. Castner

Tropical Biologist
Author
Photographer

Adjunct Professor of Biology
Pittsburg State University

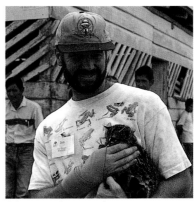

James Lee Castner was born and raised in Maplewood, New Jersey. He received his doctorate in entomology from the U. of Florida where he worked as a Scientific Photographer. An early interest in nature and insects developed into a life-long study that has led to over fifty trips to the rainforests in twelve countries of Central and South America. His study of insect biodiversity in the Peruvian Amazon has led to the discovery of over 80 new species of katydids. Dr. Castner leads workshops and tours to the tropics with Rainforest Ventures and develops educational and training materials published by Feline Press. He plans to enter secondary education as a teacher of Science and Spanish.

Stephen L. Timme

Botanist
Bryologist
Tropical Biologist

Associate Professor of Botany
Pittsburg State University

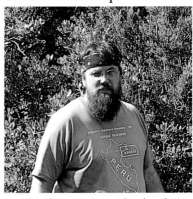

Stephen Lee Timme was born in Kansas City, Kansas, and raised nearby. He received his doctorate in Botany from Mississippi State University, after serving in Vietnam. His passion for studying and collecting plants eventually led him to the tropics and the Amazon Basin. Dr. Timme is the Vice-President for Scientific Research for the Amazon Center for Environmental Education and Research (ACEER) as well as the Director and Curator of the Theodore M. Sperry Herbarium. His book *Wildflowers Of Mississippi* is used throughout the southeastern United States. Dr. Timme leads workshops and conservation groups to the Amazon and other tropical locations with Rainforest Ventures.

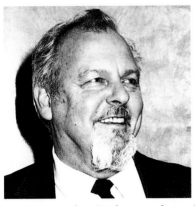

James A. Duke

Ethnobotanist
Author
Consultant

Research Botanist (Ret.) U.S.D.A.
Director, Herbal Vineyard, Inc.

   James Alan Duke was born in Birmingham, Alabama. He received his doctorate from the U. of North Carolina. After military service, he conducted ethnobotanical studies with various ethnic groups in Panama and Colombia. Much of his 30-year professional career in the USDA involved researching the cancer-fighting properties of plants. Dr. Duke has authored 20+ books on medicinal plants and traditional healing. He continues to pursue his passion for ethnobotany which has taken him all over the world. He gives lectures and classes, makes television and radio appearances, leads workshops and tours, and writes books.   He is one of the world's foremost experts on ethnobotanical uses of plants.

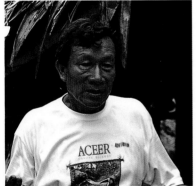

Antonio Montero

Herbal Healer
Curandero
Ayahuasquero

Curator of the ReNuPeru
Medicinal Plant Garden

   Antonio Montero Pisco was born in northern Peru and grew up in a small village along the Napo River called Kocama. At age four he went to live with his grandparents who raised him. His grandfather was a powerful shaman, and at age nine began to instruct Antonio in the arts of healing with medicinal plants and herbal remedies. Antonio continued to learn throughout his teenage years, although at times he worked for a rubber company and also in the city of Iquitos itself. He began practicing as a *curandero* over twenty years ago. He currently directs and maintains the ReNuPeru Medicinal Plant Garden which has over 160 species of medicinal and useful plants in cultivation.

Products from Feline Press

If you would like to order another copy of this book or are interested in owning other materials relating to the subjects of medicinal and useful plants, tropical fruits, hallucinogenic plants, or various other aspects of rainforest flora and fauna, please read the following.

Compact Disks (CDs)

Feline Press is currently putting together a set of CDs that will feature the plant species covered in this book, but in greater detail and with some additions. The high cost of color separations restricted the use of photographs in printed form, but much greater in-depth photographic coverage can be provided by offering the material in the form of compact disks.

Slide Sets

For those who lecture or teach classes on any of the above topics, a carousel of 35mm color transparencies is the perfect teaching aid for making a visual impact on your audience. Educators whom have neither the time nor funds to travel extensively and take their own photos can benefit from the expertise and experience of professional biologists and photographers.

Rainforest Tours, Travel, and Workshops

All of the authors lead tours and conduct workshops in their own areas of expertise on site in the tropical forests of the world. Rainforest Ventures was established in 1995 by Stephen Timme and James Castner in an effort to foster tropical conservation by making an educational trip to the Amazon an affordable reality to a wide range of people. It has been extremely successful in accomplishing this goal and both scientists now lead regularly-scheduled rainforest trips for teachers, college students, secondary students, naturalists, and tourists. For more information, contact the address below.

Feline Press
Rainforest Ventures
P.O. Box 7219
Gainesville, FL 32605

jlcastner @aol.com
sltimme@terraworld.net